Managerial Issues in
the Reformed NHS

Managerial Issues in the Reformed NHS

Edited by
M. MALEK
P. VACANI
J. RASQUINHA
P. DAVEY
University of St Andrews, Fife, Scotland

JOHN WILEY & SONS

Chichester · New York · Brisbane · Toronto · Singapore

Other Wiley Editorial Offices

John Wiley & Sons, Inc., 605 Third Avenue,
New York, NY 10158-0012, USA

Jacaranda Wiley Ltd, G.P.O. Box 859, Brisbane,
Queensland 4001, Australia

John Wiley & Sons (Canada) Ltd, 22 Worcester Road,
Rexdale, Ontario M9W 1L1, Canada

John Wiley & Sons (SEA) Pte Ltd, 37 Jalan Pemimpin #05-04,
Block B, Union Industrial Building, Singapore 2057

Library of Congress Cataloging-in-Publication Data

Managerial issues in the reformed NHS / edited by M. Malek . . . [et
al.]
    p. cm.
  Includes bibliographical references and index.
  ISBN 0 471 94033 X
  1. National Health Service (Great Britain)—Administration.
I. Malek, M. (Mo), 1949–
RA412.5.G7M36   1993
362.1'068—dc20   93–17757
                                                          CIP

British Library Cataloguing in Publication Data

A catalogue record for this book is available from the British Library

ISBN 0 471 94033 X

Produced from camera-ready copy supplied by the Editors
Printed and bound in Great Britain by Biddles Ltd, Guildford and King's Lynn

Contents

List of Contributors

Paul Beardon	*Department of Pharmacology and Clinical Pharmacology, University of Dundee*
Louise Bell	*Southend Community Care Services NHS Trust*
Reva Berman Brown	*University of Essex*
Nigel Bruce	*Department of Public Health, University of Liverpool*
Ian Cameron	*Department of Public Health Medicine, Leeds Health Authority*
Jennie Carpenter	*North Yorkshire Health Authority*
Ann-Marie Craig	*Department of Management, University of St. Andrews*
Douglas Eadie	*Department of Marketing, University of Strathclyde*
Sheila Ellwood	*Aston Business School, Aston University*
Josep Figueras	*Department of Public Health and Policy, London School of Hygiene and Tropical Medicine*
Michelle Fraser	*Newcastle Business School, University of Northumbria at Newcastle*
Brian Frost	*Management School, University of Sheffield*

Wendy Gregory   *Department of Management Systems and Sciences,*
                            University of Hull

James Harrison   *Aston Business School*

Alan Haycox   *Department of Pharmacy Policy and Practice,*
                            University of Keele

Amanda Haywood   *Department of Marketing,*
                            University of Strathclyde

Alison Henderson   *Department of Economics and Public Administration,*
                            The Nottingham Trent University

Ron Hodges   *University of Nottingham*

Elizabeth Kay   *Department of Community Medicine,*
                            University of Glasgow

Paul Kind   *Centre for Health Economics,*
                            University of York

Brenda Leese   *Centre for Health Economics,*
                            University of York

Ray Loveridge   *Aston Business School,*
                            Aston University

Mo Malek   *Department of Management,*
                            University of St Andrews

Sean McCartney   *University of Essex*

Janice McMillan   *Department of Economics and Public Administration,*
                            Nottingham Trent University

John Newton   *Newcastle Business School,*
                            University of Northumbria at Newcastle

Charles Normand   *Department of Public Health and Policy,*
                            London School of Hygiene and Tropical Medicine

Sandra Nutley   *Department of Management,*
                         University of St Andrews

Lila Pavi   *Department of Community Medicine,*
                         University of Glasgow

Joe Rasquinha   *Department of Management,*
                         University of St Andrews

Jennifer Roberts   *Department of Public Health and Policy,*
                         London School of Hygiene and Tropical Medicine

John Robinson   *Newcastle Business School,*
                         University of Northumbria at Newcastle

Geoff Royston   *Economics and Operational Research Division,*
                         Department of Health

Colin Sanderson   *Department of Public Health and Policy,*
                         London Schhol of Hygiene and Tropical Medicine

Jill Schofield   *Aston Business School,*
                         Aston University

John Sillince   *Management School,*
                         University of Sheffield

Ken Starkey   *School of Management and Finance,*
                         University of Nottingham

Sandra Subner   *Senior Scientific Officer,*
                         Camden and Islington Health Authority

Paul Vacani   *Department of Management,*
                         University of St Andrews

David Wainwright   *Newcastle Business School,*
                         University of Northumbria at Newcastle

Michael Walsh   *Department of Management Systems and Sciences,*
                         University of Hull

Acknowledgements

We wish to thank all the participants in the First International Symposium on Health Care Conference in *Strategic Issues in Health Care Management* held at the University of St Andrews, Scotland, in April 1993.

Thanks are also due to our colleagues in the PharmacoEconomics Research Centres in both Dundee and St Andrews University. We also would like to express our thanks to Verity Waite and Lucy Jepson of John Wiley and Sons, for speedy production of the book and general advice.

Finally, two very special thanks go to Deirdre Jones and Chris Evans for putting so much effort into this venture.

Mo Malek
Paul Vacani
Joe Rasquinha
Peter Davey

Preface

The organisation of health care delivery in the United Kingdom has undergone considerable change since 1989. The separation of the purchaser and provider functions has led to a massive redistribution of power and created some new centres of gravity in the process of decision making regarding allocation of secondary resources. The purpose of this book is to map out the direction in which the reforms are heading and to explore the successes and failures at both micro and macro levels. The repercussions of these reforms will inevitably be felt outside the health sector and will have profound influence on the social policy and the nature of the welfare state in the UK.

The problem with dealing with contemporary phenomena and moving targets are that one is continually in danger of basing judgement on an incomplete set of data. This is a risk which the contributors to this volume have been willing to take.

STRUCTURE OF THE BOOK

The argument surrounding the method of finance and provision of health care delivery in the western industrialised countries has always been polarised between those in favour of state provision of health care and those who put their trust in the market operation. The argument started almost immediately after the introduction of the National Health Service (N.H.S.) in Britain in 1948. F. Roberts' book on "The Cost of Health" was published in 1952 and addressed the heated argument between the pro and anti N.H.S. factions. This debate continued throughout the fifties and sixties, and went on unabated into the seventies. Although the N.H.S. underwent several reorganisations, the issue of the viability of the market relationship seemed to have died throughout this period. It re-emerged in the 1980's, first as a challenge to the highly bureaucratical managerial organisation of the N.H.S. (The Griffith Report) and then in the organisation of the method healthcare delivery itself.

This radical change raises major issues regarding accountability and governance in the new N.H.S, and is taken up by Starkey and Hodges in the first chapter of this volume. In chapter 2, Harrison and Nutley argue the case for evaluating management performance in the post reformed N.H.S. They highlight various managerial tasks that general management is expected to achieve and propose a synthetic approach to evaluation. The results of this evaluation demonstrates the varying perceptions of impact amongst the key actors and the professional groups.

In chapter 3, Schofield and Loveridge discuss the implications of the emergent hierarchical boundaries within the internal markets, the newly acquired rights and responsibilities of the GPs, and the likely impacts these may have on the provision of primary care. Primary care is also the topic of the next paper by Frost and Sillince, where a top-down planning framework is proposed to identify critical success factors needed in primary care prescribing. Robinson *et al*, in chapter 5 also report on a result of multi-disciplinary research into problems faced by the GP fundholders. The results, although tentative, are important for the policy makers and GP fundholders.

Ellwood, in chapter 6 examines the basic premises underlying market clearance in the newly created 'internal market'. In efficiently allocating factors of production, as well as consumption efficiency, prices play the important role of bringing the purchasers and providers together and facilitating transactions. Ellwood explores the costing and pricing methods of acute hospital cases in a survey of six UK hospitals and concludes with a view of how costing methods will develop as the internal market progresses.

The next two chapters are concerned with medicinal products and pharmaceutical policy. In chapter 7, Craig *et al* report the result of a survey of GPs in Scotland seeking to determine the factors influencing the prescribing behaviour of physicians. The result indicates that there are age related differentials in prescribing behaviour, implying that the younger doctors are more cost-conscious than their older colleagues. Haycox, in chapter 8 discusses the information requirement for implementing a national pharmaceutical policy and advocates a rigorous and comprehensive economic evaluation of new drugs before inclusion into the formularies. He also advocates a more active role for the government in rewarding the producers of drugs which contribute most in terms of health gain per unit of resource spent.

In chapter 9, Eadie *et al* investigate the reasons for the poor take up rate of preventative dental care in deprived areas of Glasgow. The results indicate that the problem is culturally defined rather than being service-centred. The remedy, it is suggested, is to move away from traditional treatment-oriented surgery and develop a dialogue and communication strategy reflecting the expectations of the consumer groups.

The problem of social deprivation and its link with the health status is further explored by Subner and Bruce in chapter 10. The data for this chapter comes from the electoral wards of the London Borough of Camden and Islington. The findings are not surprising as it is demonstrated that high deprivation scores are associated with high mortality and morbidity rates.

In chapter 11, Louise Bell *et al* take up the all important question of audit from the perspective of the customer and report on work in progress which aims at devising an auditing tool which is both efficient and effective.

In the next chapter, Gregory and Walsh argue that the concept of 'quality' itself is value laden and intrinsically related to the ideology. Their proposed measure of quality is also based on a dialogue between different stake holders and consensus among broad categories of the users, providers and the purchasers. Kind *et al*, in chapter 13 are also concerned with the question of quality. They report on the application of a standard psychometric scaling method applied to survey data collected from GPs in a Health Authority. The method enables GP assessments of quality to be expressed as a single index number, which in turn allowes services to be directly compared both with an average level of the Authority and a theoretical maximum value.

The reformed N.H.S. also requires a cultural change and in achieving this a re-orientation of managerial training seem to be desirable. In chapter 14, Henderson and McMillan examine the extent to which management training and development can contribute to cultural change in the N.H.S.. Their findings indicate that the contribution of formal training courses in achieving cultural change is severely constrained. In what follows they consider the policy implication of their results for the design of managed training courses for health care staff. Royston's paper, in chapter 15 deals with the development of a framework for the implementation of the National Health Strategy. He suggests a chain evaluation framework which starts from zero infrastructure and interventions, and ends with the assessment of outcomes.

The relationship between contracting and planning and its impact on the efficiency of the healthcare system is discussed by Figueras *et al* in chapter 16. They argue that based on the evidence available from the United States the effect of competition on the efficiency of the hospital sector has not been too promising. The effect of the decentralised management of the services as a by product of contracting is to increase the flexibility and reduce the barriers to change, thus helping to increase the overall efficiency of the health care system.

In chapter 17, Normand offers some thought provoking ideas. The centre piece of his conceptualisation is that changing patterns of service delivery have led to a need for more varied and diverse mixes of skills for health care professionals. This has implications for the education and training programmes of staff moving away from the current practice of enclosing staff in predetermined segments with rigid boundaries, and moving towards a training programme that helps staff to move across current professional boundaries. He argues, with some justification, that the acceptance of the current professional boundaries will not survive and those that fail to adapt will inevitably die.

Finally Malek *et al*, in a concluding postscript to the volume, outline the sources of opposition to the changes and assess the validity of the criticism laid on the reformed N.H.S. They find very little empirical evidence to support the claims of the reforms' opponents.

REFERENCES

John Jewkes and Sylvia Jewkes, The Genesis of the British National Health Service, Blackwell 1961

John Jewkes and Sylvia Jewkes, Value for Money in Medicine, Blackwell 1963.

D.S .Lees, Health Through Choice, Hobart Paper, IEA, October 1961.

Frangcon Roberts, The Cost of Health, Turnstille Press, 1952.

R.M. Titmuss, Ethics and Economics of Medical Care, Medical Care 1963.

1 Of Trusts and Markets — Accountability and Governance in the New National Health Service

KEN STARKEY & RON HODGES

University of Nottingham

INTRODUCTION

Recent years have seen the emergence of a new "discursive formation" (Preston, 1992) in health care in the U.K. The new discourse revolves around a rhetoric of markets and market relationships as an alternative to the highly structured and bureaucratised approach to organisation that has typified health provision since the inception of the National Health Service [NHS] in the period immediately after the Second World War. This new discourse and the new management structures being introduced into health care raises major issues of accountability and governance, the analysis of which, in the context of the establishment of new NHS "trusts", provides the focus of this paper.

Accountability and governance have been, in retrospect, perhaps the key issues in the evolution of management in the NHS. The dream of its founders after the Second World War was that a major infusion of resources into an integrated national health service would quickly and at one fell swoop remove the iceberg of ill health. Of course, this did not happen. Expectations of health care in the UK, as everywhere else, have continued to expand in advance of the capacity to fulfil them. Indeed, in recent years, and more particularly in the growing recessionary context of the 1980s expectations and resources, ultimately a reflection of a society's will to increase the proportion of GDP devoted to health care, have come to seem increasingly out of line with each other.

In the UK debates about accountability and governance have, historically, been dominated by the state provider's attempts to make doctors, particularly hospital consultants, more accountable to management. Doctors have framed their "refusal" to be bound by management control in terms of their clinical responsibility to the individual patient, enshrined in the Hippocratic Oath. Politicians and managers claim to be arguing for the general will when they try to make clinicians more accountable

Managerial Issues in the Reformed NHS. Edited by M.Malek, P.Vacani, J.Rasquinha & P.Davey
© 1993 John Wiley & Sons Ltd

for their resource allocation decisions. The latest attempt to make the NHS more efficient is the 1989 White Paper, and its mandate to introduce more market-like processes into the relationship between purchaser and provider of health services, in particular the establishment of trust status for various medical units and budget-holding status for general practices.

ORGANISATION DESIGN, ACCOUNTABILITY AND THE NHS

The major attempts to make the NHS more accountable have emphasised structural change in the various reorganisations that have marked the Service since its inception. One can briefly summarise the legacy of these structural changes up until the last White Paper as bureaucracy in the hospital sector and independent contracting in primary care. General medical practitioners (GPs) have jealously guarded their independent status but this has been at the cost of a degree of marginalisation and diminished power over resource allocation when compared with the powerful hospital consultant groups. Hospital consultants "bought" into the NHS earlier than GPs. In Aneurin Bevan's famous phrase when asked how he gained their complicity in the setting up of the NHS when GPs continued to resist, "I stuffed their mouths with gold", thus effectively silencing their objections.

Hospitals have been the major users of NHS resources and consultants and their interest groups, particularly the powerful Royal Colleges, have played a central role in recourse allocation decisions, frequently through their ability to resist change and safeguard the *status quo*. As a result resource distribution patterns have tended to be dominated by professional aspirations and the extension of past service patterns. Consultants have resisted the emergence of alternative policy agendas aimed at radical reorganisation. *Plus ca change, plus c'est la meme chose* (Clark & Starkey, 1988)! Critics of the medical profession, as represented primarily by hospital consultants argue that exacerbating the problem of scarce resources is the profession's inability and unwillingness to come to terms with notions of general interest based on the managerial values of efficiency, accountability and economy (Haywood & Alaszewski, 1980). The most important weakness of the NHS that has prevented any coherent attack on the problem of improving resource usage has been the persistent failure to develop a form of governance that reconciles the interests of clinicians and managers of the service. The medical profession's notion of clinical freedom exacerbates the problem which has been further worsened by "the long chain of responsibility stretching from Parliament and the Secretary of State to the doctor and nurse at the patient's bedside" (BMJ, 1985: 132).

Earlier reorganisation of the NHS, in particular the major 1974 reorganisation, focused on centralisation, hierarchical structures and tightly defined managerial roles in the light of centrally defined policies. This coined the famous phrase "delegation downwards should be matched with accountability upwards" (Alaszewski *et al.*, 1981: 4). With the advice of American management consultant, McKinsey & Co., structural solutions and mechanistic systems of management were emphasised at the expense of more organic, flexible forms. Clinicians were to be incorporated into the managerial process through representation on the key decision-making bodies. The aim was to replace political-incremental "decision drift" with rational managerial decision-making and to reverse the "policy drift" to high technology medicine dominated by the hospitals and the acute medical specialities. Under the new "Cogwheel" structures introduced after 1974 and based on the principle of consensus management clinicians found the endless time needed for management meetings particularly irksome and a distraction from what they considered their major role, clinical medicine. Consensus in these management meetings proved very difficult to achieve and implementation even more difficult! Of course, the excuse of lack of time for not doing certain kinds of work can actually demonstrate a lack of commitment to that work (Marks, 1977).

The medical profession tends to define the problems in the NHS solely in terms of scarce resources.

> The medical profession therefore escape all blame for the shortcomings of the service and virtually remove from the agenda all examination of how existing resources are used or misused. Governments, the Treasury, the DHSS [now the Department of Health] become the villains to be blamed. The central problem of clinical freedom and resources remains safely off the agenda (Wilding, 1982: 30).

The profession demands that the public accepts on trust its implicit responsibility while the paymaster has increasingly demanded "explicit public accounting" and accountability. The starting point for the influential Griffiths Report of 1983 was that the weakness of the NHS stemmed from a lack of a clearly defined management function covering planning and performance appraisal - Griffiths "suggests that most of the weaknesses in NHS management - imprecise objectives, little measurement of health output, infrequent evaluation of performance against agreed clinical, social and economic criteria - flow from this general organisation defect" (House of Commons Social Service Committee, 1984: 179). As the Report so graphically expressed it, if Florence Nightingale used her lamp to search out NHS managers, even she would have a hard task finding those with explicit managerial responsibility for much NHS work and outcomes. This invisibility and powerlessness of management raised major problems of accountability.

Griffiths recommended general management as the means of providing the managerial control and leadership that the NHS has historically lacked. The Report also stressed the need for acceptance by clinicians that the allocation of resources is related "to priority needs in the population and to some acceptable level of cost and effectiveness" (NHS Management Inquiry, 1983: 130). The profession was urged to come to terms with the limits on clinical autonomy that are implicit in finite resources:

> "The most critical issue of all is the sense among clinicians that there is pressure on resources, that they cannot expect any radical change for the better, and that as a consequence of this realisation they develop cooperative rather than competitive modes of behaviour" (NHS Management Inquiry, 1983: 130)

in their negotiations about resource allocation. The injunction is that clinicians frame their resource demands in terms of a notion of accountability to the general will not just to their own specialism. They are required to think holistically not functionally.

Griffiths also constitutes an explicit argument for the introduction of a private sector rationality into the public sector.

> We have been told that the NHS is different from business in management terms, not least because the NHS is not concerned with the profit motive and must be judged by wider social standards which cannot be measured. These differences can be greatly overstated. The clear similarities between NHS management and business management are much more important. In many organisations, in the private sector, profit does not immediately impinge on large numbers of managers below Board level. They are concerned with levels of service, quality of product, meeting budgets, cost improvement, productivity, motivating and rewarding staff, research and development, and the long-term viability of the undertaking. All things that Parliament is urging on the NHS. In the private sector the results in all these areas would normally be carefully monitored against pre-determined standards and objectives (NHS Management Inquiry, 1983: 10).

Its chairman's managerial expertise and reputation had been gained in the retail sector with supermarket giant Sainsbury.

It is useful here to situate the issue of NHS management and the proper balance of managerial and clinical inputs into decision-making in the context of more general debates about professionals and managerial control. The concept of professionalism can be used by a profession as "a strategy for controlling practice" (Esland, 1980: 340) and as political ploy in the bargaining process over work definition and independent status in an attempt to protect professional autonomy. But the use of the notion of professionalism as a device to distance an occupational group from external accountability is increasingly criticised. We have seen the growing use of more explicit performance indicators in a variety of professional contexts, exemplified by moves to closed contracts (Starkey, 1989). In medicine, in the USA, the medical insurers have been powerful, as the ultimate reimburser of medical fees, in introducing medical audit, specifying limits to the amount of expenditure they will reimburse for the treatment of particular disease entities, a move criticised as leading to "cook book medicine" by some doctors. In the U.K. we have the Korner initiative aimed at specifying norms for health care provision on a variety of parameters. A major problem that the proponents of the use of such indicators have to resolve is that indicative pricing might have unintended consequences for some "marginal" client groups, thus actually restricting access to medical care for those who need it most. In the chilling warning of the British Medical Association, "If productivity were the yard-stick, consultants would invariably avoid the difficult case, the special need, to treat the quick case, involving the minimum trouble, with the most certain outcome and the quickest discharge" (BMA, 1982).

ACCOUNTABILITY TO PATIENTS

The 1989 White Paper "Working for patients" took as its basic premise that *all* hospitals and GP practices need to be raised to the level of the best.

New management information systems have provided clear evidence of a wide variation in performance up and down the country. In 1986-87, the average cost of treating acute hospital in-patients varied by as much as 50 per cent between different health authorities, even after allowing for the complexity and mix of cases. Similarly, a patient who waits several years for an operation in one place may get that same operation within a few weeks in another. There are wide variations in the drug prescribing habits of GPs, and in some places drug costs are nearly twice as high per head of population as in others. And, at the extremes, there is a twenty-fold variation in the rate at which GPs refer patients to hospital.

The White Paper set two objectives:

i.   to give all patients better health care and greater choice of services
ii. and, to reward NHS staff who successfully responded to local needs.

To achieve these ends various key measures were suggested including:

- *more delegation to the local level* with responsibilities delegated from Regions to Districts and from Districts to hospitals to make the service more responsive at the local level;
- *self-governing hospitals* — hospital trusts with more freedom to take the decisions which most affect them, such as determining their own pay levels and borrowing money;
- *GP practice budgets* — GP practices free to use their budgets as they see fit in contracting for services from various providers;
- *new funding arrangements* so that money goes directly to where the work is done best;
- *better audit arrangements* — more rigorous auditing of quality of service and value for money, with the extension of "medical audit" by peer review throughout the NHS.

The White Paper ruled out any radical change in the basis of funding for national health care. Mrs. Thatcher, herself, recalling her defensive statement of 1982 that the NHS was safe in Conservative hands, said in the Foreword that the NHS would continue to be available to all, regardless of income, and to be financed "mainly out of general taxation". Consideration had been given to alternative funding mechanisms, such as expanded private insurance schemes, but studies repeatedly demonstrated that the British system, "which places the Treasury in a strategic position to police annual increases in NHS revenues", is "by some distance" the cheapest means of funding comprehensive access to health care, a fact reflected in the relative levels of GDP various nations devote to health care (Holliday, 1992). But the White Paper was radical in its suggestions concerning NHS management and organisation, primarily in its suggestions concerning the introduction of an internal market in health care services based upon the allocation of separate purchaser-provider roles among various agents and agencies.

Most radical of all the ideas arising from the White Paper was the creation of new types of purchaser and provider — GP fundholding practices and NHS trusts. (At first trusts referred to hospital but their remit has grown in other ancillary services such as ambulances.) The fundholding practice contracts for its own health services. The non-fundholding practice has its purchasing performed by its agent, the District Health authority (DHA). The fundholding practice is thus free to "shop around" for best value services for its patients. Under this regime the GP is to act as patient's "advocate". The DHA continues to act for the fundholding practice on bills for service beyond a certain financial limit, thus protecting fundholding practices from potential moral hazard and financial problems of excessive expenditure, in a situation of fixed budgets, on any one patient.

It is envisaged that by 1993 25% of the population will be registered with a fundholding practice. It is also estimated that by then 200,000 beds, more than two-thirds of the total, will be in trust hospitals (Holliday, 1992). The logic of these changes is that a market for health services will impose a market discipline on providers such as trusts, force them into rational pricing decisions and drive down costs as providers compete on the grounds of efficiency. Competition will be in terms of price and quality of care. Resources will follow the decisions of purchasers. There will also be competition for patients among purchasers who will have to make the services they offer, their own care services as well as their purchasing decisions, attractive to potential patient-clients.

THE ATTRACTIONS OF TRUST STATUS

Content analysis of hospital applications for trust status allows us to see how providers of care are responding to these measures and to see if their expressed rationale for seeking trust status corresponds to the philosophy of the White Paper. We examined twenty three applications documents of second and third wave trusts based in the Trent Regional Health Authority, 10 general hospitals, six community care units, three mental handicap units, two special hospitals and two ambulance services, a reasonably representative spread of activities. We also examined the annual reports and accounts of 55 of the 57 first wave trusts which covered the year ending 31st of March 1992 to see what their actual experiences of trust status were.

The most commonly mentioned reason for moving to trust status is the benefit to patients. Emphasis is on responsibility to local purchasers of services. Examples include "plans to develop new complementary services and to improve existing services". Trust status would "help us to set our priorities in collaboration with patients, general practitioners and the (local) Health Authority". In some cases specific examples are given, for example, "to provide an acute hospital to the East of the county". Mission statements reflect this emphasis on the provision of services in a local market for care, for example "...the provision of comprehensive, high quality, efficient mental health and community health services which are, as far as possible, locally based and sensitive to local needs." The other continuous theme in all of the applications we have read is the generation and maintenance of quality with many explicit references to quality measurement and audit.

FREEDOM TO MANAGE

"Freedom to manage" is another explicit theme throughout the documents.

> We would be able to look at our problems and solve them without having to wait for decisions from District or Regional level. For instance, it would be possible to set our own targets for waiting times, to arrange community transport schemes or to make changes to catering services to allow patients more choice.

> At present the way in which the NHS is managed is very complex, several tiers of management are involved with policy making which in turn affects the time scale in which the Service can respond to change. [As an NHS Trust we will be] operationally independent and [this] will facilitate faster decision making at a local level.

FINANCIAL CONTROL

The financial control rationale of applying for trust status is clearly put in the following:

> It is unlikely that, as a Directly Managed Unit, the District would be able to support a maintenance or a capital programme of the size required. However as an NHS Trust we will be able to retain depreciation and any other surplus we make to maintain the building and replace old and worn out assets. In addition, we will have the flexibility to borrow extra money to supplement internally generated funds.

The importance of being commercially minded was implicit in all of the statements. "Profit-making" is an increasing managerial concern involving a reappraisal of trusts' business "portfolios":

> "... a group will get together in the near future to look at income generation schemes specific to Priority Care Services, moving the action away from Acute Services where money making ideas have been centred in the past."

MANAGEMENT STRUCTURES

Management structures are a crucial factor in establishing the governance relationships of any organisation. The new structures proposed in trust applications are all very similar because of Department of Health guidance specifying the need for non-executive directors and four of the executive posts. There is some feeling among trusts that this guidance "restricts the range of managerial skills that can be adequately represented at Board level." A common way around this problem was to create an Executive Management Board or team with a wider range of skills which them reported to the Trust Board. Other arrangements included:

i.   Appointing a Commercial Director reporting to the Board through the Chief Executive;

ii.   Appointing a sixth executive director to the Trust Board such as a Director of Estates;

iii. Having a Personnel Director not on the Board but reporting directly to it.

The composition of a first wave Trust Boards is summarised in Table 1.

Table 1. Composition of First Wave NHS Trust Boards as given in Annual Reports.

	TOTAL	MALE	FEMALE	NOT GIVEN (note 1)
Chairperson	55	53	2	
Non-executive Directors	238	167	71	
Chief Executive	54	49	5	
Nursing Director	39	5	34	
Medical / Clinical Directors	54	36	8	10
Finance / Information Director	49	43	6	
Personnel / Human Resources	25	19	6	
Director of Operations	16	11	5	
Director of Support Services	5	5	0	
Director of Hospital Services	3	2	1	
Director of Corporate Affairs or Organisational Development	8	6	2	
Research & Development	6	4	0	2

Note 1: These figures indicate those circumstances when the title given in the Annual Report (Professor, Doctor) did not indicate whether the office holder was male or female

Note 2: In those circumstances where more than one person had held any particular office during the year the figures above represent the person in office at the date of publication of the Annual Report.

Note 3: There were 55 Annual Reports available for this survey. The holder of the Chair was indicated in all cases, the Chief Executive in 54 instances, and other directors in 50 instances.

A number of points of interest emerge from this table. The absence of an explicit Director of Personnel or Human Resources is noteworthy given the White Paper emphasis on lacal responsibility for staffing matters including, perhaps, local pay bargaining. It appears that personnel matters are not considered as a senior management role. Very few women appear on the boards yet women are the majority of NHS employees and trust application documents emphasise equal opportunituies policies. A predominance of non-medically qualified staff is also noticeable. The combination of four or five non-executive directors together with a chief executive and a finance director in most cases exceeds the number of medical specialists!

STAKEHOLDER ANALYSIS

A stakeholder is any group or individual who can affect, or is affected by, the achievement of a corporation's purpose.

Stakeholders include employees, customers, suppliers, stockholders, banks, environmentalists, government and other groups who can help or hurt the corporation. The stakeholder concept provides a new way of thinking about strategic management -that is, how a corporation can and should set and implement direction (Freeman, 1984).

According to stakeholder analysis organisations are stronger to the extent that they demonstrate a broad sense of responsibility to a variety of stakeholders, both external and internal. Trust applications stress the role of staff as stakeholders. Trust status brings with it local responsibility for attracting and retaining staff. The applications also focus on accountability to other stakeholders. Local voluntary groups are often mentioned, although little specific detail is given. One exception is the following:

"As a Trust we would wish to develop and nurture these friendships so that members of the [specific] support groups continue to feel a part of the Trust's future."

Detail is then given of the work of seven support groups. Ethnic minorities and equal opportunities are also stressed, for example:

"The hospital is currently reviewing all its written information in conjunction with local ethnic community leaders to take into account their social and cultural needs. An interpreter service is currently being developed in outpatients...".

Other service providers are mentioned as being strategically linked to trusts such as other local hospitals. There are various examples of hospitals in the same geographical area stating that they will continue to work together to provide complimentary services. This recalls the emphasis in the recent literature on organisation design (Miles & Snow, 1986) that networks will form a dominant organisational and transaction mode for future business. Judkins and West (1985) argue that systems need to be designed, with the aid of new information technology, to provide lateral, horizontal, multidirectional and even overlapping linkages to facilitate the flexibility of organisations. In the NHS developments in information technology have a crucial role to play in making the new system work as they will be the source of information on such crucial factors as pricing, waiting times and quality of service.

Recent strategic management literature has frequently linked stakeholder analysis to the organisation's sense of mission. NHS trust mission statements are framed in terms of a missions that stress a range of stakeholders and differing definitions of social responsibility. Compare the following mission statements:

(A) We are committed to provide high quality and standards of treatment, care and support - to the population served by the Trust.

(B) Our mission is to provide prompt, personal clinical care and promote the health of those served by the [Trust]. We will continue to advance as a centre of excellence in patient care, teaching and research ...

(C)   The five Units [combining to pursue trust status] are determined ...to:

- put patients and their carers first by sensible and close cooperation across a wide range of services;
- work closely with ... other relevant organisations to ensure a successful and strong base for teaching and research ...
- work together to promote high quality employment practices, with an emphasis on equal opportunities and a wide range of staff development and rotational training opportunities;
- avoid wasteful competition in services where this would divert resources from the care of ... patients.

Mission (C) presents a clear sense of the complexity its new status will occasion. It is also framed in terms of a sense of accountability to a broad range of stakeholders - patients, carers, allied organisations, staff. Missions (A) and (B) are narrower/more focused. Mission (C) also raises explicitly what must be a major issue in the new internal market for health resources - wasteful competition. We turn to this issue next when we consider trusts' accountability to District Health Authorities and Regional Health Authorities.

ACCOUNTABILITY AND STRUCTURE

One of the guiding principles of the 1989 White Paper is that "Delegation downwards must be matched by accountability upwards". General managers, the "children" of Griffiths, are already formally accountable for the spending of their units. The White Paper seeks to make doctors more accountable. The White Paper proposed an NHS Management Executive to be responsible for all operational matters. However, given the impossibility of the Executive exercising effective authority over the 190 District Health Authorities (DHAs), Regional Health Authorities (RHAs) were to continue to ensure that Government policies, the province of the new NHS Policy Board, chaired and appointed by the Secretary of State for Health, are properly carried out within their Regions. The White Paper defines essential tasks for RHAs as including: setting performance criteria, monitoring the performance of the Heath Service and evaluating its effectiveness. As for the DHAs, the establishment of self-governing trusts is premised on the principle that there is scope for delegating decision-making from DHAs to trusts. The Government objective is to create organisations in which those who are actually providing the services are also responsible for day-to-day decisions about operational matters. Trusts are also concerned with strategic matters relating to their own long-term goals. In this context the role of the District is problematic. The White Paper states, that having devolved operational control, DHAs, like RHAs,

can then concentrate on ensuring that the health needs of the population for which they are responsible are met; that there are effective services for the prevention and control of diseases and the promotion of health; that their population has access to a comprehensive range of high quality, value for money services; and on setting targets for monitoring the performance of those management units for which they continue to have responsibility.

This monitoring role is particularly problematic. Figure 1 sets out the new management structure of the NHS.

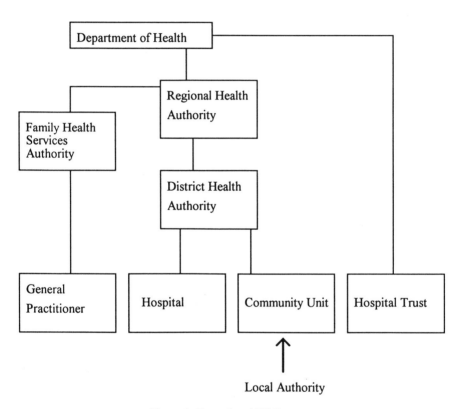

Figure 1. Post-reform NHS Structure
Source: Whynes (1992)

If the philosophy of the White Paper becomes reality we will see increasing numbers of quasi-independent hospital trusts directly responsible to the Department of Health. GP practices which opt for budget-holding status will receive their budgets directly from the Regional Health Authority but the FHSA which has replaced the Family Practitioner Committee will continue to hold their contracts and be responsible for monitoring expenditure against budgets. In this scenario the role of the DHA as an important purchaser of services and "champion of the people" (Department of Health, 1990) seems increasingly marginal. Indeed, the role of Region is also problematic as its direct responsibilities seem to veer more towards general practice as hospitals opt for trust status! The principle of devolution of authority downwards leaves unclear the relative reponsiblities over the longer term of RHAs, DHAs and FHSAs. Indeed, speculation is rife in the NHS about mergers between FHSAs and DHAs and their is considerable debate about the commissioning (service planning and development) role of FHSAs (a role also supposed to be done at the more "macro" level by Regions) and the purchasing role of DHAs. The purchaser roles of RHAs and DHAs must logically shrink.

It has been suggested that DHAs and RHAs are likely to take on entirely new roles under the new structure and to act as local and regional regulators in a decentralised NHS (Holliday, 1992: 71). Regions will monitor issues of specialisation in particular services in their area, investment infrastructure, and illogical choices at too local a level, for example, the duplication of services. RHAs would seem to be well placed to perform this task of regulation. For DHAs, currently involved in the purchasing role which the logic of the reforms dictates they will cede to GP fundholding practices, the future is more problematic. It is GP fundholders who will become increasingly responsible for health needs assessment and the pattern of local service contracting.

ACCOUNTABILITY TO GENERAL PRACTITIONERS

One decoding of the White Paper from a political point of view is in terms of the relationship between the providers of primary and hospital care. The GP and community care has frequently been seen as a "Cinderella" area of the NHS when it comes to funding. One can attribute a political agenda to the White Paper - that it represents an attempt to swing the balance of power back form the consultant to the GP. The GP under the new arrangements has a potentially crucial role as contractor for and purchaser of services that hospitals will provide. The GP thus assumes an important new role of gatekeeper, a role they have always to some extent played in their hospital referral capacity but now the difference is that they have the power to "shop around" in an internal NHS market among providers and to judge provision in terms of value for money -what price is being asked for what surgical procedures, for example? - and in terms of waiting time. GPs thus have a much more powerful role as patient's advocate and judge of the relative merits of providers, their medical peers in many cases when they are assessing the relative merits of hospitals for patient referral purposes. GPs who manage their own budgets will be looking to maximise their benefits in contracting for service. This makes hospital accountability to GPs a key issue.

In practice, to judge from the trust annual reports, this new role for GPs is as yet under-developed. The proportion of income from GP fundholders in these hospitals was typically very low (See Table 2). However trust documents express explicitly the expectation that the proportion of income from general practice fundholders will increase significantly in the year's ahead as the fundholding scheme is extended to more practices, for example:

We are investing in our Financial Plan in new information technology links to General Practitioners..... We are developing joint Patient Satisfaction Surveys with local GP practices and in 1992/93 are piloting reference groups on our services as part of our approach to improving quality , centred on GP surgeries..... We have a City First Digest which all GP Fundholders receive, giving information bi-monthly on changes in our services and prices. City First, the monthly magazine for Derby City General Hospital, is sent to all GPs in Derbyshire.

We will seek to develop personal understanding of our services through personal contact....holding Open Days.....Contract Reviews and our GP hotline......and move towards our staff providing services in GP premises.

According to the view from the FHSA the introduction of the new 1990 GP contract was designed to promote a shift from a relatively exclusive pre-occupation with the individual doctor-patient relationship in general practice to a broader practice population focus, and from a preoccupation with treating illness to a concern for preventing illness and promoting health. The new Contract also envisaged "the linking of remuneration, increased GP accountability, more consumerism, and the intended introduction of competition between practices. ... GPs [are to be] held responsible for the provision of specified information, and of hours, times and types of service that would have been unthinkable just a few years ago" (Yorkshire Health Authority, 1991) Despite the rhetoric it is, as yet, unclear how FHSAs will actually manage GP fundholder's supposed new accountability. On the one hand budgetary devolution is announced, on the other a new accountability is introduced via contract and competition!

Table 2. Sources of Total Income of 53 First Wave Trusts

	£ millions	%
Health Authorities	2,363.6	87.7
GP Fundholders	29.0	1.1
NHS Trusts	4.5	0.2
Department of Health	21.3	0.8
Private Patients	30.8	1.1
Other	5.7	0.2
Patient Transport Services	5.4	0.2
Other Operating Income	225.1	8.4
Charitable Donations	3.4	0.1
Transfers from Donation Reserve	5.9	0.2
TOTAL	2,694.7	100

CONCLUSION

Of course, the NHS is not alone in having to deal with the problems of control and coordination in the large organisation. Because of its size, however, and the professional nature of key employees who have traditionally seen autonomy as an essential element of their employment contract, one sees these problems writ large. It is interesting to situate the changes in NHS in the context of the broader picture of corporate restructuring that is emerging in other sectors and in the context of the analysis of management and transaction costs. Coase (1937) examined the conditions in which internal organisation is preferable to market transactions. The firm was seen as a means of reducing transaction costs. Chandler's (1977) seminal study of the growth of managerialism traces a major transition in organizational governance from the invisible hand of the market to the visible hand of the managerial cadre. One of the main arguments for internalisation of activities and vertical integration according to transaction cost theory is that it permits the firm to economise on the cost of negotiating many separate market contracts (Williamson & Ouchi, 1981: 348-50). However, various internal control problems can lead to a reassessment of internalisation (Wright, 1988). Alternative modes of organizing, market or quasi-market, may be deemed more efficient in terms of their ability to economise on transaction costs. There are limits to the efficiency and effectiveness of bureaucracy. Firms "grow until the marginal cost of discovering opportunities for gain within the firm exceeds the marginal cost of discovering opportunities for gain in the market" (Johnson & Kaplan, 1987: 88).

Increasingly we are witnessing a return to market or quasi-market transaction modes. Current changes in the NHS are premised on the efficacy of internal market contracting between independent providers competing for the contracts that will guarantee their viability. NHS plc under the new regime, if it does emerge, will be a very different organisational animal than the bureaucratic monolith the White Paper seeks to sweep aside. In the literature on corporate restructuring and changes in ownership form arising from the markets and hierarchies perspective we see the same emphasis on the dysfunctional consequences of large-scale bureaucratic organization (Starkey, 1991). Changes in ownership form are seen as a major means of resolving the tension between management and ownership. Again, the changes in the NHS seem to be imbued with some of this logic. The newly emerging independent trusts and fundholding general practices are to be given back ownership of their own destiny.

What we see in the 1989 White Paper and the applications for trust status under the NHS's new managerial regime is an agenda for change. We will have to wait for the Annual Reports of later wave trusts and the development of GP fund-holders to see if this agenda develops in the way the White Paper anticipates. We will also have to wait until the new managerial regime governing the relationships of trusts, fundholding practices, RHAs, DHAs, FHSAs and the Secretary of State for Health emerges in which the relative responsibilities of these parties becomes clearer. Neither the White Paper nor subsequent Working Papers clearly explain the reason for retaining RHAs or the nature of regional control of DHAs, FHSAs and self-governing trusts (Kinston, 1989: 110). In the interim the various providers and purchasers vie for continuing legitimacy and power.

According to the view from the FHSA the introduction of the new 1990 GP contract was designed to promote a shift from a relatively exclusive pre-occupation with the individual doctor-patient relationship in general practice to a broader practice population focus, and from a preoccupation with treating illness to a concern for preventing illness and promoting health and the FHSA has a crucial role to plat in this. The new Contract also envisaged "the linking of remuneration, increased GP accountability, more consumerism, and the intended introduction of competition between practices. ... GPs [are to be] held responsible for the provision of specified information, and of hours, times and types of service that would have been unthinkable just a few years ago" (Yorkshire Health Authority, 1991) Despite the rhetoric it is, as yet, unclear how FHSAs will actually manage GP fundholder's supposed new accountability. On the one hand budgetary devolution is announced, on the other a new accountability is introduced via contract and competition!

The Region also seeks clarification of its role.

> The Secretary of State is expected to retain wide reserve powers and is likely to use them for political reasons or at the behest of the Treasury to block competitive ploys or operating tactics or pricing techniques of the type routinely employed by businesses to attract custom and gain a business advantage. The RHA (who else?) will surely be expected to monitor and exercise control on his behalf (Kinston, 1989: 110).

There is much uncertainty, confusion and legitimate concern about the future. Markets have replaced planning as the principle driver of resource-allocation. The new principles are in place, a new discourse has emerged. Practice is more problematic.

REFERENCES

Alaszewski, A., Tether, P. & McDonnell, H. (1981) "Another dose of managerialism? Commentary on the Consultative Paper 'Patients First', *Social Science and Medicine*, 15A, 3-15.

British Medical Association (1982) "Evidence to DDRB [Review Body on Doctors' and Dentists' Remuneration", London, British Medical Association mimeo.

Chandler, A.D. (1977) *The Visible Hand. The Managerial Revolution in American Business* Cambridge MA, Bellknap Press.

Clark, P. & Starkey, K. (1988) *Organization Transitions and Innovation-Design* London, Pinter Publishers.

Coase, R.H. (1937) "The nature of the firm", *Economica*, 4, 386-405.

Esland, G. (1980) "Professionals and professionalism" in G. Esland & G. Salaman (eds) *The Politics of Work and Occupation,* Milton Keynes, Open University Press.

Freeman, R.H. (1984) *Strategic Management. A Stakeholder Approach,* Boston, Pitman.

Haywood, S. & Alaszewski, A. (1980) *Crisis in the Health Services* London, Croom Helm.

Holliday, I. (1992) *The NHS Transformed* Manchester, Baseline Books.

House of Commons Social Services Committee (1984) "Griffiths NHS Management Inquiry Report", London, HMSO.

Johnson, H.T. & Kaplan, R.S. (1987) *Relevance Lost* Cambridge MA, Harvard University Press.

Judkins, P. & West, D. (1985) *Networking in Organisations* Aldershot, Gower.

Kinston, W. (1989) "The role of the Region in the post-White Paper NHS", *Health Services Management,* June, 110-113.

Marks, S.R. (1977) "Multiple roles and role strain: some notes on human energy, time and commitment", *American Sociological Review,* 42, 921-936.

Miles, R.E. & Snow, C.C. (1986) "Organizations: new concepts for new forms", *California Management Review,* 28, 3, 62-73.

National Health Service Management Inquiry (1983) "Report", London, DHSS.

Preston, A.M. (1992) "The birth of clinical accounting: a study of the emergence and transformations of discourses on costs and practices of accounting in U.S. hospitals" , *Accounting, Organizations and Society,* 17, 63-100.

Starkey, K. (1989) "Time and professionalism: disputes concerning the nature of contract", *British Journal of Industrial Relations,* XXVII, 375-396.

Starkey, K., Wright, M. & Thompson, M. (1991) "Flexibility, hierarchy, markets", *British Journal of Management,* 2, 165-176.

Whynes, D. K. (1991) "Economic perspectives on the National Health reforms", *Economics,* XXVII, Part 3, No. 115, 108-112.

Wilding, P. (1982) *Professional Power and Social Welfare* London, Routledge & Kegan Paul.

Williamson, O.E. & Ouchi, W.G. (1981) "The markets and hierarchies and visible hand perspectives" in A.H. Van de Ven & W.F. Joyce (eds) *Perspectives on Organization Design and Behavior* Chichester, Wiley.

"Working for Patients" (1989) London, HMSO.

Yorkshire Health Authority (1991) "FHSAs ... Today's and Tomorrow's Priorities" mimeo.

2 Whither Health Service Management?

JAMES HARRISON[1] **& SANDRA NUTLEY**[2]

[1]*Aston Business School*
[2]*University of St Andrews*

INTRODUCTION

It is only relatively recently that the word management and people with the titles of managers have come into widespread use in the public sector. Public administration has been replaced by public sector management. There are multiple reasons for this shift from administration to management and, as Hood (1991) points out, these are likely to involve a series of political, economic and social factors. The oil crises of the 1970s coupled with the growing concern about the increase in public expenditure are undoubtedly major factors. In addition, in both the British National Health Service (NHS) and local government there has been a concern to exert greater control over professionals' expansion of their services.

In Britain, particularly under the Thatcher government, a series of initiatives were introduced to address these concerns. Taken together they are characterised by Hood (ibid) as a "new public management" doctrine, a doctrine which is by no means unique to Britain. Hood (ibid, pp 4-5) highlights seven key elements of this doctrine:

- hands on professional management in the public sector;
- explicit standards and measures of performance;
- greater emphasis on output controls;
- shift to disaggregation of units in the public sector;
- shift to greater competition in the public sector;
- stress on private sector styles of management practice;
- stress on greater discipline and parsimony in resource use.

Much of this doctrine rests on importing private solutions to public sector problems and several writers have commented on the difficulties associated with this conceptualisation. Firstly, there is some doubt about whether there is a set of standardised prescriptions on managerial competencies and practices which applies across private, let alone public, sector organisations (Willcocks and Harrow, 1992). Secondly, there is the question of the extent to which the public sector is different to

Managerial Issues in the Reformed NHS. Edited by M.Malek, P.Vacani, J.Rasquinha & P.Davey
© 1993 John Wiley & Sons Ltd

the private sector and hence requires different managerial skills and practices (Allison, 1979; Smith Ring and Perry, 1985; Ranson and Stewart, 1989). Specifically focusing on health services, both Weisbrod (1976) and Klein (1985) have emphasised some of the unique factors of health care which limit the extent to which knowledge developed in a commercial environment can be transferred into the management of health services. Pollitt (1990) argues that, in any case, the managerial solutions being imported are an impoverished concept of management. Does this mean that management and the public sector do not mix? Gunn (1988) argues not, saying that what is needed is a third way; the what and why of public administration are distinctive, but the how can be drawn from business practice.

Traditionally, management in the NHS was characterised by consensus, involving the heads of the different service areas. Consensus management, however, fell into disrepair. During the 1970s the Service became increasingly bureaucratic and unable to adapt to changing circumstances. In addition, its costs grew dramatically and despite efforts to contain these and refashion the organisation in 1974 and 1982, expectation and dissatisfaction mounted.

Harrison *et al* (1989b) report that between the late 1960s and 1982 there were some 25 empirical research projects focused on the management of the NHS. The main findings of these studies were that the NHS was not a unitary organisation in which managers were the major source of influence. Professionals dominated, particularly the medical profession. Management was characterised as reactive rather than proactive, change was incremental with only marginal impact upon the status quo. Management activity was considered to be producer oriented. Harrison et al (ibid) conclude that the pre-1982 management culture was that of diplomacy where managers acted as maintainers.

Between 1982 and 1984 a number of initiatives were introduced in an attempt to address the above problems. These included the requirement to identify efficiency savings, the introduction and reporting of performance indicators, cost improvement programmes, and competitive tendering for hospital support services. It was against this backdrop that the NHS Management Inquiry was established by Norman Fowler (the then Secretary of State for Health and Social Security) in February 1983, and chaired by Roy Griffiths, a prominent businessman. The result of the enquiry was "to review current initiatives to improve the efficiency of the health service in England and to advise on the management action needed to secure the best value for money and the best possible service to patients" (Fowler, 1983). The principal recommendations of the Inquiry report concerned:

- The creation of an NHS Supervisory Board and a Management Board to provide a central management focus.
- The creation of a general management function. Health Authority chairmen were required to identify general managers, clarify the role of chief officers and review and reduce functional management.
- Greater prominence and priority for the personnel and property functions.
- The streamlining of consultation procedures.

- The need to seek out and respond to the views of the consumer/ community and to use these views in shaping policy and monitoring performance. (NHS Management Inquiry, 1983).

The second half of what soon became known as the Griffiths Report set out some of the reasoning behind the recommendations:

- individual overall management accountability could not be located.
- the machinery of implementation was generally weak.
- a lack of orientation towards performance in the service.
- a lack of concern with the views of consumers of health services.

Griffiths saw the way forward inextricably linked to the creation of general management which he defined as "the responsibility drawn together in one person at different levels of the organisation for planning, implementation and control of performance" (NHS Management Inquiry, 1983: 11).

Arguably the Griffiths Inquiry potentially addressed items 1, 2, 4 and 6 of Hood's list (above). The extent to which it actually addressed these issues will be considered in the remainder of the paper. Whilst the NHS was still in the process of making a reality of general management, a new initiative was launched with the Working for Patients White Paper (1989); which developed into the NHS and Community Care Act 1990. This legislation primarily focused on creating an internal market for health care services and can be seen as introducing items 3, 5 and 7 of Hood's list into the NHS.

This paper will argue that the Working for Patients legislation should be seen as complementary to, rather than as a substitute for, the general management initiative. We should not see the internal market as removing the need to be concerned with management performance. Indeed, the need for successful general management is even more pressing following the Working for Patients reforms, which came into effect in April 1991. Despite this, relatively little has been done to evaluate general management as a policy initiative. Such evaluation is important in its own right as well as forming a necessary part of considering the present capacity of health service management.

The first part of this paper explores in greater detail what general management was intended to achieve and the various ways in which it has been conceptualised. It also summarises the findings of existing research in this area. A case study of general management in one district health authority during the period 1987 to 1992 is then provided. The final section of the paper provides a postscript covering the period 1989 to 1992. It also draws out conclusions in terms of the managerial performance which will be a pre-condition for sound financial performance and survival in the context of the NHS reforms introduced in 1991.

UNDERSTANDING GENERAL MANAGEMENT — DEFINITIONS AND EVALUATIONS

Defining General Management

The Griffiths Report argued that general managers were to create the conditions in which the meta objective of the best possible service to patients could be realised. Thus although general management was defined in terms of individual action, it was also implicitly defined as an end state organisational condition. In this sense Griffiths saw general management as both means and ends. Subsequently, throughout the literature, general management is almost simultaneously used as both verb and adjective. At times general management is viewed as a set of behaviours and at other times as a particular management genre or culture (for example, see IHSM, 1985 and IHSM, 1987). The existence of the former being necessary to create the conditions for the latter.

The ambiguity emerging when attempting to define the nature of general management makes an evaluation of it somewhat difficult. Hunter and Williamson (1989) raise five key issues regarding the nature and evaluation of general management:

- what is precisely meant by general management in the NHS;
- the extent to which general management has remained true to the principles set out in the Griffiths Report;
- the extent to which general management meant different things in different authorities/ countries;
- the extent to which the direction of the NHS is the result of general management or the influence of financing, performance review or increased central direction;
- the extent to which it has been practical and feasible to involve clinicians in management.

Thus there is an acknowledgement of differing definitions across authorities and the problem of disentangling the effects of general management from the many other factors influencing the direction of the NHS.

Evaluating General Management

Whilst it seems self evident that important and costly programmes be evaluated to determine their effectiveness, this is a comparatively recent phenomenon in the UK. By contrast there is a much stronger record of policy evaluation in the USA. There have been attempts to evaluate the general management initiative and these are considered below.

It is possible to visualise the general management initiative and the research associated with it in terms of a systems model where inputs are converted into outputs (see figure 1). In terms of evaluation it is possible to add outcomes; that is, the impact of the outputs produced. Using this model, evaluative research can focus on the extent to which the intended inputs are put in place. It can also look at the process by which these inputs are converted into outputs. Finally, it can consider the outputs from such a process and/or the outcomes from the system as a whole. This multi-layered nature of evaluation is reflected by Herman *et al* (1991) who distinguishes between organisation review, formative and summative evaluation, implementation and outcome studies.

Another important dimension in evaluative research is the extent to which it focuses on description — telling things as they are — or whether its focus is normative — telling things as they should be.

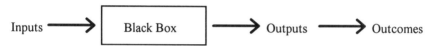

Figure 1. System representation of inputs converion to outputs

The literature concerned with the input component of the systems model has been concerned with the extent to which the infrastructure of general management has been put in place. A number of studies have, as part of their research brief, considered the nature of the infrastructure established under general management (Banyard, 1988a & 1988b; Harrison et al, 1989b). The conclusions from this research is that there are some commonalities amongst the infrastructural arrangements established under general management, but there are also differences which reflect the varying ways in which general management has been interpreted. The normative side of this literature has been concerned to identify the optimum conditions under which general management could be established and flourish (Dearden, 1985; Stewart and Smith, 1988)

The black box is the least understood element of the model. Attempts to throw light on the conversion of inputs to outputs are dominated by practitioner experience which is richly diverse but of variable quality. Babour (1989), Wall (1989) and Nicholls (1989), as Unit General Manager, District General Manager and Regional General Manager respectively, describe "the view from the trenches". Their views on process tend to be concerned with judgements upon personal or situational success. Whilst this adds colour and texture to the literature, generally, it offers little in terms of rigour or explanatory substance. "For the moment , notions of success remain elusive and imperfectly understood by general managers" (Babour, 1989, p 56).

The literature focusing on the output side of the systems model is largely concerned with the products of general management and its success or otherwise. One study in this area (Allaway, 1987) is a study of failure, another (Strong and Robinson, 1988) is a study of the philosophy, rationale and initial impact of general management. This latter study is important as one of the earliest attempts at evaluation with a multi-district focus.

There are several contributions which are concerned with tracing the impact of general management on specific functional areas within the NHS — the impact of general management upon finance (McNally, 1985), capital planning (Harvey, 1987) , and medical autonomy (Harrison, 1988; Harrison et al, 1989a). These tend to see general management simply as an influence upon a given task environment rather than as either a pattern of managerial behaviour or as a new environment.

An evaluation of outputs and outcomes raises the important issue of the criteria to be adopted in such an evaluation. Best (1987) argues that any evaluation of general management should be concerned with the extent to which:

• there is access to the service
• provision is relevant
• provision is effective
• equity can be demonstrated
• the service is socially acceptable
• service is conducted with due efficiency and economy

Alternatively, Davies (1988) suggests three criteria:

• is decision making speedier than before?
• how far do general managers favour resource management as a means of influencing medical staff?
• how far has general management led to a more consumer orientated service?

The former criteria are concerned with the outcomes of the Service under general management. The latter more closely follows the contours of Griffiths' own definition and thinking about the outputs of general management.

However, even the identification of intermediate outputs (as opposed to outcomes) is not straightforward - "it is easier to point to progress in managerial change than to output or outcome achievements" (Stewart and Dopson, 1987: 444). Accordingly, some studies have focused on the general managers themselves in an attempt to shed light on both the "black box" and some of the effects of the managerial activity observed. Perhaps the best known such study is the Templeton Series, a "tracer study" of 20 district general managers between April 1985 and September 1987. The project, under the direction of Rosemary Stewart, published its findings in nine reports. Report No. 8 compared the achievements of general management with expectations (NHSTA, 1987). Encouragement was drawn from a bias for action, the breaking down of inappropriate professional barriers, involving doctors in management and influencing clinical practice, improvements in the measurement of health output, devolution, and improving the sensitivity of the service to the consumer. The authors were, however, careful to qualify these findings in the following terms:

• the difficulty of knowing how much would have been accomplished without reorganisation;
• implementation of general management was accompanied by a financial squeeze.

- the short elapse time between adoption and implementation;
- the need to rely upon the respondents' accounts of progress;
- the difficulty of measuring outcomes;
- the different manner in which district general managers fulfilled their role.

These qualifications are an important reminder that the systems model outlined above should not be seen as a closed system. Factors other than the inputs of general management influence the processes within the black box and the outputs achieved.

Another important contribution to bridging the gap between the process of general management and its effects is the study carried out in various units throughout Trent and North East Thames RHAs. The study concentrated on general management at unit level and consisted of interviews with unit general managers and the completion of questionnaires by a sample of unit staff (Banyard, 1988). The study identifies key areas of success and problem areas: decision-making was considered to be quicker and communication improved, but the medical profession still remained independent and the impact of general management at first line level was perceived to be slight. The study concluded that a small majority (53%) regard unit general management overall as having been a favourable innovation.

The most extensive study on the outputs and to some extent the outcomes of general management is that conducted by Harrison et al (1989b). They interviewed some 400 people in eight English health districts and two Scottish health boards during the period Spring 1987 to Autumn 1988. They consider the respondents' views on how well some of the specific changes associated with general management were working out in practice. What they find is a variation of views between professional groups and between levels within the NHS. To take just a few examples:

- Decision making was considered to be speedier by about half of the senior managers. Nursing staff were the most convinced of this and consultants the least convinced.
- There was a perception of a greater clarity of roles, with a more precise allocation of personal responsibility. However, it was believed that this greater clarity did not extend down the hierarchy beyond unit general managers.
- All the authorities studied had spent a large slice of time on structural arrangements, but their was a great variety in local structures.
- There was widespread cynicism as to whether a greater consumer responsiveness had developed.
- There was a widespread use of performance indicators, but this was more evident amongst planning and finance staff than amongst medical or nursing staff.
- On the whole it was felt that "management stops at the consulting door" (ibid. p. 10) and that doctors, in general, do not concede the legitimacy of anything other than a diplomatic (maintenance) model of management.

Their key research question is whether there has been a cultural shift in the NHS following the implementation of the Griffiths Report. They conclude that "such attitudinal changes as have taken place cannot be said to add up to a major cultural shift" (ibid. p. 15). On the whole the Harrison et al study is less optimistic about the outputs and outcomes of general management five years after its introduction than some of the earlier studies. A variation in outputs is noted, but the process by which these outputs were achieved is still little understood.

A CASE STUDY OF GENERAL MANAGEMENT

One thing that is clear from the literature on general management is its potential to have a profound influence upon the NHS. The research reported in this part of the paper was born out of a desire to explore in detail the extent to which this potential has been realised. The research began in 1988, five years after the Griffiths Report. At this time there had been relatively few attempts to evaluate the impact of general management.

The research site for this evaluation was an urban district health authority (DHA) serving a population of 240,000 with a budget of £54m. It was decided to focus on a single authority in order to give detailed consideration to the implementation and effects of general management. The choice of this particular setting was influenced by the fact that one of the authors worked there and hence had greater access to information than might otherwise have been achieved. The data on the implementation and effects of general management was collected in two phases, by two different methodologies. The first phase of participant observation was authorised by the District Management Team in April 1988 and a report on this phase of the research was presented to the District General Manager in 1989. In addition to the internal researcher gathering information by participating and observing, this phase of the research was informed by numerous internal reports, documents, and written correspondence. In order to obtain a wider view of the perceptions of the success or otherwise of the general management initiative in the DHA, the participant observation phase was followed by a systematic survey of the senior managers of the DHA during 1989. A postal questionnaire was used to obtain the views of:

- the whole of the District Management Board (14 people, including each of the unit general managers)
- the accountant, estates manager and personnel officer based in each unit
- the director, nurse manager and administrator of each of the ten service programmes.

In total 49 people were approached and 48 of these responded.

It is possible to group the recommendations of the Management Inquiry under three headings (see below). These headings were used to collect information on the implementation of general management in the DHA in question and they are also used to structure the presentation of the results in this section of the paper. They are concerned with identifying the inputs of general management and its intermediate outputs.

The establishment of the infrastructure	— appointment of general managers — creation of a management structure — revision of functional management
The establishment of supporting/reinforcing systems	— extension of the review process — revised decision-making process — improved budgeting arrangements — involvement of clinicians in management
The promotion of a corporate/strategic focus	— to the management of human (personnel) and material (estates) resources — to the notion of environmental exchange via consultation, interaction and quality

The results from both of the research phases are reported below, first by considering the phase one participant observation, and then by looking at the questionnaire results.

Results of phase one — participant observation

The establishment of the infrastructure

The infrastructure established in this DHA followed the proposals developed by the District General Manager (DGM), which were published in an internal report in 1985. The structure, at first glance, followed a familiar pattern of grouping services and institutions into units, and heading each of these units with a Unit General Manager (UGM). A closer examination reveals a more complex structure; the proposals aimed to blend the devolution of management responsibilities to units with a programme structure which sought to identify clear responsibility for developing programmes of care for particular client groups. The resulting organisational structure is illustrated in Figure 2. It consists of three management units (in addition to the central headquarters) and ten programme areas (each headed by a programme director).

There was a major change in functional management responsibilities. No longer was there a line management relationship between the functional officers based in the units and their former superiors based in the District Head Quarters (DHQ). All nursing and estates personnel became accountable to their respective UGM

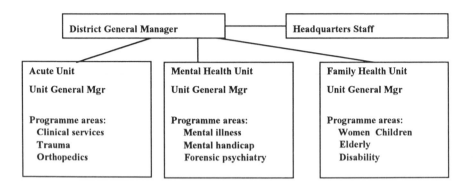

Figure 2. Organisational Structure of the District Health Authority

overnight. Similarly, the outposted finance and personnel specialists became operationally accountable to their UGM. The new arrangements were akin to a matrix structure, with all the potential benefits and attendant problems that this might entail (Davis and Lawrence, 1977). Although programme areas were, organisationally, located within units, their remit entailed that they look at services on a district wide basis.

It was left to the newly appointed UGMs to breath life into the structure, and they did so in highly individualistic ways, resulting in a lack of uniformity across the district. As more and more responsibilities were devolved to units, the DHQ became more uncertain of its role. As the financial situation deteriorated, the DHQ was initially seen as a potentially unnecessary overhead and then, as more difficult choices had to be made, as being unable to provide a coherent overall view or sense of direction.

There was little preparation for the infrastructure changes which were implemented. Whilst the changes themselves were publicised, there was no comprehensive organisational development programme. It was not until November 1987 that a Director of Organisational Development was appointed, and November 1988 before the Personnel Department published a training strategy. The changes to the line management of functions appeared to have a profound effect on nursing and estates staff who both felt they had lost control of their profession and that their influence had been significantly reduced. The result of these changes was characterised as resulting in anomie for nursing staff and anarchy for estates staff.

The establishment of supporting/reinforcing systems

The establishment of key supporting systems were also envisaged in the DGM's proposals. The extension of the review process was linked to the creation of a new central directorate concerned with policy, direction and performance management. Whilst decentralisation and a central performance management focus are not mutually exclusive, the failure to make explicit the latter's relationship to the former contributed to an initial sense of unease and persistent tension in central/local relationships. Progress was made on monitoring performance, but this was not matched in terms of policy analysis and development. Policy tended to be interpreted as "what we can do" and hence performance measurement focused on what was done, rather than what should have been done.

The new management structure itself was intended to achieve and reflect devolved decision-making. There was indeed a shift from a predominantly central pattern to one which was a mixture of central and local decision-making. It is worth distinguishing between operational and strategic decision-making. In specific and discrete terms, operational decision-making appeared to be more speedy and sensitive to local needs. However, this was almost always at the expense of an authority-wide consistent approach to operational issues and working practices.

Strategic decision-making proved more problematic. Such responsibility formally lay with the District Management Team (later extended and renamed the District Management Board — DMB). However, internal reports described this team as "not a corporate body, more an aggregate". There were a variety of attempts to establish an overall strategic direction: a Strategic Overview (1986), an Environmental Analysis (1987) and a Business Plan (1988). Despite these attempts, corporate management remained illusive and problematic. Matters came to a head during the autumn of 1988 when the DMB was unable to reach an agreed view upon the financial situation. The two day retreat organised to consider this crisis concluded that there was no coherent or shared strategic direction, low strategic control and instability.

In the absence of a shared sense of strategic direction, units developed largely incrementally and in response to operational issues. Boards had been established at unit level, as well as at district level. Whilst the Acute Unit Board acted as a board and met frequently, the Family Services Unit Board met much less frequently and almost under pressure, the Mental Health Unit Board seldom met and persisted in refusing to see itself as more than the sum of its parts.

Part of the drive towards improving budgetary arrangements was to devolve some financial management responsibility to units and support these units by outposting management accountants to them. The budget structures moved from being geographical/functional to being generic/unit budgets. Within these units budgets, assets and resources were then allocated to the relevant programme areas. The budget structures remained somewhat notional; the way in which they were configured was not always consistent with the expectations of the Department of Health or the Regional Health Authority, and they were not truly representative or controllable in programmatic form.

Following a national trend, there were attempts to place the responsibility for budgetary control in the hands of those who committed the expenditure (i.e. the clinicians), but progress was very slow. There were also moves to involve clinicians (doctors and nurses) in the management of services. Of the ten programme director posts, eight were occupied by clinicians (and five of these were doctors). However, whilst clinicians were involved in management, the nature of that involvement was more apparent than real. With regard to the doctors occupying programme director posts:

- their accountability to general management was in terms of their part-time management role rather than as clinicians
- their role with regard to their respective programmes was one of providing "programme leadership" together with "clinical integrity and direction" rather than exercising conventional managerial control
- whatever the precise definition, the authority they exercised - particularly with regard to their peers — was by consent.

The promotion of a Corporate/Strategic Focus

To some extent the existence (or otherwise) of a corporate/ strategic focus has been discussed under the heading of improved decision-making. On a more general level, senior managers were identified as being "failure avoiders" rather than "success seekers" and the short term tended to drive out the long term.

The Griffiths Report emphasised the benefits to be derived from managing personnel and estates assets corporately. The DGM's proposals tended to emphasise the former rather than the latter. Even with personnel, it was several years (after the implementation of general management) before a strategic direction was provided in terms of personnel policy and training, and coherent staff planning remained a distant prospect. A formal review of estates was not completed until September 1988 and then there was only slow progress in implementing the review's findings.

The last area to be considered under the strategic heading is described as environmental exchange; that is, the consultation and interaction with the community at large, including the pursuit of excellence in the form of quality assurance. Paradoxically, whilst the authority developed a strong emphasis on marketing itself to the community, its record on formal consultation was patchy, and there was unease at working with the Community Health Council and voluntary groups.

In summary, the recommendations emanating from the NHS Management Inquiry anticipated greater directional clarity, improved decision-making and (more) effective implementation of policies. The participant observation phase shed doubts on the extent to which these outputs had been achieved. Much had been changed in the DHA in question, but the benefits of these changes were not yet readily apparent.

Results of phase two — the questionnaire survey

The questionnaire was designed around the same three areas of:
- infrastructure
- supporting/reinforcing systems
- corporate/strategic focus

In addition questions were asked about how respondents viewed the overall outcome of general management.

Table 1. Questionnaire Survey Statements

The implementation of General Management has resulted in —

1. general managers each with a personal responsibility for their Unit/ District
2. a clear identity for their Units/ Districts.
3. people in all the clinical disciplines making an important contribution to the management an delivery of services.
4. a legitimate concern with performance.
5. the devolution of decision making.
6. budget setting being shaped by workload consideration.
7. the professions playing a substantial part in the running of services.
8. the District as a whole sharing a common purpose.
9. a consumer orientation in the provision of care.
10. general managers having more of an impact upon decisions effecting patient care.
11. the presence of clear leadership.
12. a Unit/ Programme structure which is superior to the previous organisational pattern
13. the management role of Nurses remaining undiminished.
14. a review process concerned with evaluating outputs and outcomes in order to facilitate service delivery.
15. speedier decision making.
16. general managers being more involved in setting budgets and allocating resources than managers were in the past.
17. the greater involvement of clinicians in management via the Programme Director role.
18. the pursuit of a systematically developed and clear District strategy.
19. the pursuit of excellence via quality enhancement programmes and related methods.
20. benefits to the organisation as a whole.
21. a concern on the part of a general managers with only his Unit or District.
22. a clear understanding on the part of staff as to how the organisation is structured.
23. the management role of the Estates function remaining undiminished.
24. a review process mainly concerned with exercising central control.
25. an improvement in communication throughout the organisation.
26. an improvement in budgetary matters as a result of better information/ the existence of Unit Accountants.
27. Resource Management as the (financial) means of controlling the Medical profession.
28. the District as a whole being more that the sum of its "four Units".
29. a desire on the part of the District as a whole to work with/ influence key groups within the community at large.
30. benefits in the care and treatment of patients.
31. the organisation, on the whole, being better managed.

In order to achieve both a high response rate and obtain a consistent set of data, the questionnaire was highly structured and designed for quick completion. Respondents were asked about the extent to which they agreed with particular statements. A five point Likert scale was used to structure their responses (on a scale from strongly agree to strongly disagree). The statements are listed in Table 1. Table 2 shows how these statements relate to the recommendations and anticipated consequences of the NHS Management Inquiry. Figures 3 and 4 show the level of respondents agreement with each of the statements. The main points to emerge from their responses and the extent to which they diverge from the conclusions of the phase one participant observation are highlighted below.

Overall, the picture emerging from phase two of the research is more positive than that emerging from phase one. This could, in part, be due to the fact that phase two occurred one year later than phase one and things may have improved during this intervening period. More likely it reflects the differing methodologies and the danger during participant observation of being overly influenced by negative signals, together with the potential problem of questionnaire respondents answering questions in the way in which they think they should be answered.

Table 2. The relationship of the survey statements to the recommendations and expected consequences of the NHS Management Inquiry

		Statement Nos.
Infrastructure	Appointment of General Managers	1, 11, 21
	Organisational Structure	2, 12,22
	Functional Management	3, 13, 23
Supporting systems	The Review Process	4, 14, 24
	Decision Making	5, 15, 25
	Budgetary matters	6, 16, 26
	Participation of clinician and other professionals	7,17, 27
Corporate/Strategic focus	Corporatism	8, 18, 28
	Environmental exchange	9, 19, 29
Outcomes	Patient services	10, 20, 30

Despite an overall positive impression to emerge from the phase two survey, there were areas where general management was not seen as delivering the expected goods and the areas of concern reflected those highlighted in phase one. In general the most strongly supported statements relate to general management resulting in better services (outcomes). This is followed by support for statements suggesting that the new infrastructural arrangements have produced internal benefits. The least supported statements relate to the existence of a corporate/strategic focus and the existence of effective support systems. Just over 60% of respondents thought that the district as a whole was sharing a common purpose and nearly as many thought that a clear district strategy was being pursued. In retrospect, an important survey result was that only about 30% of respondents thought that the budget setting process was now shaped by workload consideration and only just under a half thought that budgetary information had improved.

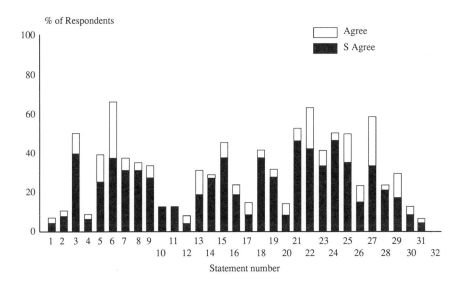

Figure 3. Percentage of Respondents Disagreeing with Questionnaire Statements on General Management

As would be expected there were variations across the organisation. DHQ staff were generally more positive in their evaluation of general management than others. Surprisingly, the Acute Unit (the one unit identified as acting as a unit) were the most negative. The Acute Unit were sceptical about the organisation's structure, the role of programme directors, and were the most unconvinced group regarding the contribution of clinicians and the value of quality enhancement programmes. Generally, nursing and estates office staff were less positive about general management than other professional groups.

POSTSCRIPT AND CONCLUSIONS

The existing research on evaluating the general management initiative paints a somewhat variable picture. Early optimism is in contrast to later scepticism. Reasonably consistent findings revolve around:

- speedier decision making
- more devolution of managerial responsibilities
- greater concern with performance measurement
- greater clarity of roles
- more of a consumer orientation

The case study reported here echoes some of these findings and also amplifies them. Whilst decisions were felt to be speedier, these tended to be decisions on those

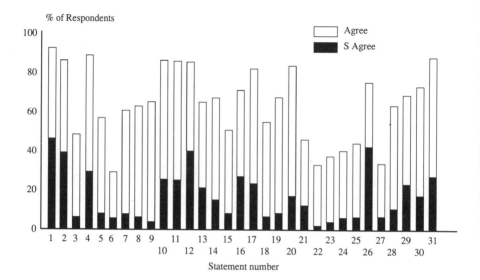

Figure 4. Percentage of Respondents Agreeing with Questionnaire Statements on General
Management

operational matters which had been devolved to unit level. The price for this increase
in speed was greater diversity in operational practices across the DHA.
Improvements in strategic planning and decision making proved more difficult to
achieve. There was a danger of strategy remaining at the level of slogans. Central
policy and performance review structures could be accused of colluding with this
approach in focusing on monitoring what was done, rather than what should have
been done. One of the reasons for the lack of progress on strategy was the difficulty
of getting to grips with some tough resource allocation decisions. The inappropriate
budget structures and the lack of appropriate financial and activity information was a
block to effective decision making. The benefit of greater clarity of roles resulting
from the general management initiative was clouded in the case study DHA by the
matrix structure which resulted in some confusion and a potentially "two-hatted" role
for programme directors as they faced the new initiative of the internal market.
There appeared to be a loss of clarity or justification for the role of the DHQ and
central — local relationships were tense and contentious. The units may have been
clearer about their role but they had difficulty in considering themselves as more than
the sum of their parts. Finally, the greater consumer orientation was in danger of
being one-sided — telling the consumer more, but not necessarily listening to what
they had to say in return.

The way in which the above findings and concerns were manifest in the subsequent experience of the case study DHA is considered below.

Postscript — 1989 to 1992

The period 1989 to 1991 in the case study DHA was dominated by planning and preparation for the implementation of the Working for Patients (WfP) reforms. This preparation was made all the more complex by first the threat and then the reality of a merger between the DHA and one of its neighbours. The merger eventually occurred in April 1991 (at the same time that the WfP reforms came into operation!). The structure of the DHA up to this point remained relatively stable in terms of the number of units and the cross-cutting programmes.

During the period March to October 1990 a trial run at operating within the internal market was approved (after some initial reticence and obstruction) and undertaken. The early temptation for potential purchasers and providers to retreat into their respective corners was resisted. A maxim to emerge almost from the outset was that "we must work together so that we might work apart". The trial threw up familiar problems of the lack of information, the lack of shared understanding and some skills deficiencies. Whilst it generally achieved its learning objectives, it failed in respect of being able to price the contracts arrived at. One of the dilemmas addressed was the role of the programme directors. Initially it was thought that they would become the purchasers for their programme area. This proved difficult given the conflict of interest with their strong service delivery orientation. Instead it was decided that in the majority of cases their role needed to become more managerially focused within provider units.

The merger with the neighbouring DHA resulted in some (now) ten units being refashioned into five new units (each with its own UGM). Programme directors in some places remained, some were retitled/ refocused, but most such posts simply disappeared. The matrix structure, as a consequence, also disappeared and was replaced by "local centralism" as devolution progressed.

Units initially tried to assert their independence in the wake of the WfP White Paper. However, as the complexity of the tasks facing them started to emerge they began to sink some of their historical differences and work more closely together. The financial crisis (see below) at first reinforced the need to work together, but subsequently the large acute unit began to dominate the organisational landscape. All units are now progressing trust applications, early interest having been discouraged by the RHA for "strategic" reasons. It remains to be seen whether this apparent harmony between units will survive as local competitive forces grow.

Very soon after the merger to form a large purchasing authority, the developing financial difficulties burgeoned into a £30m+ shortfall crisis. Whilst financial problems inevitably attend the merger of two deficit authorities, and the cost of the merger itself and the simultaneous establishment of the internal market undoubtedly exacerbated underlying difficulties, the scale of the problem was unparalleled. Why should this be so? Much was made of the inherited nature of the problem and, in some measure, this may offer a partial explanation. However, the time taken to uncover the problem (circa 7 months), to adequately define it (approximately a further 6 months) and for the RHA's patience to be finally exhausted with progress towards resolution (some 6 months more) are all consistent with continuing difficulties in respect of decision making and budgetary matters. These difficulties were a continuing theme in both phases of the research and a feature of the pre-implementation trials. They are concerned with the allocation of resources and thus lie at the very heart of the management process.

Conclusions

Interesting as the above vignette is, to what extent is a concern with general management and the performance of general managers still of relevance? Despite the elapse time since its implementation and the WfP reforms, general managers still hold sway as the chief executives of purchasing authorities and as the leaders of directly managed units/ NHS trusts. As such the leadership cadre of the NHS is central to its operations and future. In a post-reform world purchasers will need more than ever to demonstrate stewardship over increasingly large sums of public money and to exercise careful choice and wise investment. This will be important for the health and well being of all those on whose behalf they procure health provision. By the same token, providers will need to understand and control costs in order to set and manage prices within the internal market. In short, speedy and effective decision making and competent financial management will be of critical importance to the health expectation of whole communities and to the viability and survival of trusts.

If it is reasonable to assume that general management is still relevant under different circumstance, is it the same general management as earlier defined? The short answer is yes, but altered circumstances will inevitably bring about shifts in emphasis. Given, for example, the introduction of market mechanisms, the notion of customer orientation, important in 1983, is fundamental in 1993. Units will have to look to the interests of their customers, i.e. purchasers, who in turn will have to be sensitive to their customers, i.e. their immediate community. Another example is the participation of clinicians. Whilst this might be described as an emergent issue in 1983, it is central to the implementation of resource management and the establishment of clinical directorates in 1993. A decade in time, similar dimensions, but some difference of meaning.

The greatest difference however, is likely to be observed in the form and manner of general management leadership. Originally conceived of as a managerial elite, general managers were highly individualistic and the source of a personal vision of the future. To what extent does this remain the case? In terms of regional and district health authorities, general managers and other senior managerial figures have, as a consequence of reform, been incorporated as executive *members* of their authorities. Whilst they will remain full time professional managers, unlike their part time lay non-executive colleagues, the dynamic will, or at least should, change. Whilst managers will still have to account for their performance, matters of policy and direction should increasingly be issues for the Board as a whole. No longer can members blame officers, or officers scapegoat members! Equally, as units become self-governing trusts, Boards will be formed of a size and nature similar to those in nearby DHAs. Whilst these changes may appear to be the same, their impact will be proportionately greater in Trust settings since unit general managers have enjoyed a degree of freedom and independence not found elsewhere in the NHS. The role of purchaser and provider organisations may be increasingly divergent but the models for their direction and control are converging. The model of the company board and corporate governance is the obvious analogue. In such a setting executives and non-executives will increasingly concern themselves with questions of direction, accountability, executive management and supervision. The extent to which such changes can take root and, if so, be successful, will be critical to the success of the reforms and to the future of the NHS. This will establish a further agenda in respect of the evaluation and development of health policy.

REFERENCES

Alleway, L. (1987), 'Back on the outside looking in', *The Health Service Journal*, 16th July, 818-819

Allison, G.T. (1979), 'Public and private management: are they fundamentally alike in all unimportant respects?', Public Management Research Conference Paper, Brookings Institution, Washington DC (Reprinted in Perry, J.L. and Kraemer, K.L. (eds) (1983), *Public Management: Private and Public Perspectives*, Mayfield Press, California)

Banyard, R. (1988a), 'How do UGMs Perform', *The Health Service Journal*, 21st July, 824-825

Banyard, R. (1988b), 'Watching the Revolution', *The Health Service Journal*, 11th August, 916-917

Barbour, J. (1989), 'Notions of "Success" in General Management', *Health Services Management Research*, 1(1), 53-57

Best, G. (1987), *The future of NHS general management: where next?*, King Edward's Hospital Fund for London, London

Davies, P. (1988), "More than just window dressing", *The Health Service Journal*, 14th July, 790-791

Davis, S.M. and Lawrence P.R. (1987), *Matrix*, Addison-Wesley, London

Dearden, R.W. (1985), 'The Development of General Management', *Hospital and Health Service Review*, July, 163-164

Fowler, N. (1983), *Statement on the NHS Management Inquiry*, Department of Health and Social Security, London, 26th October

Gunn, L. (1988), 'Public Management: a third approach', *Public Money and Management*, 8 (1&2), 21-25

Harrison, S. (1988), *Managing the NHS: Shifting the Frontier?*, Chapman & Hall, London

Harrison, S., Hunter, D.J., Marnoch, G. and Pollitt, C. (1989a), 'General Management and Medical Autonomy in the NHS', *Health Services Management Research*, 2(1), 38-46

Harrison, S., Hunter, D.J., Marnoch, G. and Pollitt, C. (1989b), *General Management in the NHS: Before and After the White Paper*, Nuffield Institute, University of Leeds, Leeds

Harvey, D. (1987a), 'The Impact of General Management', *Public Finance and Accountancy*, July, 8-10

Harvey, D. (1987b), 'The Impact of General Management', *Public Finance and Accountancy*, July, 13-16

Herman, J.L., Morris, L.L. and Fitz-Gibbon, C.T. (1991), *Evaluator's Handbook*, Sage, London

Hood, C. (1991), 'A public management for all seasons?', *Public Administration*, 69, 3-19

Hunter, D.J. and Williamson, P. (1989), 'Perspectives on General Management in the NHS', *Health Service Management Research*, 2(1) 2-9

IHSM (1985), *NHS General Management: Implementation*, Institute of Health Services Management, London

IHSM (1987), 'Memorandum to the Social Services Select Committee', *Hospital and Health Service Review*, July 177-178

Klein, R. (1985), 'Management in health care: the politics of innovation', *International Journal of Health Planning and Management*, 1, 57-63

NHS Management Inquiry (1983), *Report* ('The Griffiths Report'), Department of Health and Social Security, London

NHSTA (1987), Templeton Series on DGMs, directed by Rosemary Stewart, Issue Study No. 8, *Role and Progress of DGMs: An Overview*, National Health Service Training Authority, Bristol

Nicholls, R.M. (1989), 'Central-Local Relationships in the Aftermath of Griffiths', *Health Services Management Research*, 2(1), 58-63

Pollitt C. (1991), *Managerialism and the Public Services: the Anglo-American Experience*, Blackwell, Oxford

Ranson, S. and Stewart, J. (1989), 'Citizenship and government: the challenge for management in the public domain', *Political Studies*, 37 (1), 5-24

Secretaries of State for Health, Wales, Northern Ireland and Scotland (1989), *Working for Patients*, CM555, HMSO, London

Smith Ring, D and Perry, J.L. (1985), 'Strategic management in public and private organisations: implications of distinctive contexts and constraints', *Academy of Management Review*, 10 (2), 13-19

Stewart, R. and Smith, P. (1988), 'Lessons for Managers', *The Health Service Journal*, 21st January, 90

Strong, P. and Robinson, J. (1988), *New model management: Griffiths and the NHS*, University of Warwick, Warwick

Wall, A. (1989), 'Griffiths Five Years On', *Health Services Management Research*, 2(1), 47-52

Weisbrod, M. (1976), 'Why organisational development hasn't worked (so far) in Medical Centres', HMC Review, cited in Pettigrew, A. et. al. (1988), 'Understanding Change in the NHS', *Public Administration*, 66, 297-317

Willcocks, L. and Harrow, J. (eds) (1992), *Rediscovering Public Services Management*, McGraw-Hill, London

3 Markets or Hierarchies?
Top Down or Bottom Up Reform of
Primary Care Delivery in the NHS?

RAY LOVERIDGE & JILL SCHOFIELD

Aston Business School

The reforms to the NHS introduced in the 1990 Act were designed to give considerable managerial responsibility to GPs as "users" of a variety of secondary resources. In practice managers in FHSAs have taken the initiative in shaping the strategic parameters within which GPs exercise their new-found discretion. With hindsight it can be seen that FHSA management were likely to play a major part in the reshaping of the heterogeneous array of statutory and voluntary contributors to primary care and to the creation of new links with secondary carers.

Given the artisanal nature of GP employment it might also be seen that the realisation by GPs of their ability to exercise market leverage in a formative way would be slow to manifest itself. This paper will examine a number of recent reports of GP responses to their new rights and responsibilities and raise questions about the emergent hierarchical boundaries to the internal market within which these are likely to be exercised by GPs.

THE NEW PUBLIC MANAGEMENT

Over the period of sustained, if uneven, economic expansion experienced by all Western capitalist countries after World War II aspirations for increased levels of publicly provided services among citizens of those countries appear to have grown even more quickly. This is especially true of health care where the proportion of an expanding Gross Domestic Product that all Western nations spend on medicine has itself increased significantly. Small wonder then that an apparent levelling off in the economic expansion of these countries over the latter part of the 1970s brought about an almost universal concern for containment of public expenditure and for more effective monitoring of the public provision of services.

This concern took three forms:

Managerial Issues in the Reformed NHS. Edited by M.Malek, P.Vacani, J.Rasquinha & P.Davey
© 1993 John Wiley & Sons Ltd

i.   Attempts to slow down or reverse the growth in public expenditure and public indebtedness. These latter have subsequently proven extremely resilient to political interest. In the USA under the Reagan Administrations and in the UK under Thatcher public expenditure actually increased and reliance in public indebtedness could be seen as gaining in strategic significance as the manufacturing bases for direct value added activity collapsed in both countries (Dertouzos *et al*: 1990).

ii.   The establishment of central performance assessment systems for the monitoring and appraisal of the use of publicly provided resources. Resource management rather than administration was to be appraised. The change in terminology implied a devolution of more authority to operational level. Modes of Scientific Management were to be adopted as means to achieve the declared goals of economy, efficiency and effectiveness. (Bovaird *et al* 1991).

iii. A shift towards privatisation and quasi-privatisation in which core government agencies adopted a "facilitating" role in respect to the contracting out the provision of services to private providers rather than providing them "internally" through direct employment.

This concern for the establishment of greater central control over the provision of public services can be seen to date back, at least, to the 1970s (Bovaird *et al* 1991). Its expression in the loosely-linked modes of devolved management described as New Public Management (NPM) in Rhodes (1991) might be attributed to three main factors. The first was the regeneration of liberal doctrines such as contestability, user choice and transparency in both academic theory and in public rhetoric (Hood: 1990). The second was the creation of unemployment on a scale that enabled policy makers to mount market based assaults on institutionalised interests in a climate that was conducive to the imposition of radical changes (Pirie: 1988). A third, and somewhat paradoxical trend, was seen to be toward greater consumer discrimination and desire for novelty. Whether representative of a fundamental change in personal expectations as suggested in Post Modern, Post-Industrial meta-theories or simply a rational response to depressed markets, the adoption of consumer rights as a major plank of most political parties in the West ensured its formal salience in NPM rhetoric.

A fourth factor to which some significance has been attached by analysts has been the increasing availability of information technology (IT). This has been seen as providing opportunities for both integrating and standardising the systemic provision of strategic and operational information (Child and Loveridge: 1990). Beyond the purely managerial use of IT, its application in the NHS was pioneered by clinical diagnosis and treatment. In the managerial sphere however, we are inclined to see the impact of IT as being that of enabling change rather than being a factor in causing the movement to NPM.

Critics of NPM, such as Pollitt *et al* (1990) suggest that across a wide range of principal agencies an emphasis on cost saving and the importance attributed to financial measures of performance has led to a neglect of effectiveness and emphasis on short term managerial definitions of economy and efficiency. In periodic value-for-money appraisals it is difficult to include end-user opinion on effective value. Even in qualitative analyses provided by external consultants such as that of Pettigrew *et al* (1992) the success of organisational change does not appear to have been judged against any direct end-user (patient) evaluation. Indeed Pollitt *et al* report members of district and unit management groups as describing consumer initiatives as "glib", "cosmetic" and even "bullshit" (Pettigrew *et al*, 1992: 68)

Another criticism has been directed at the underlying doctrine leading to a belief in the superiority of market relationships over hierarchically imposed means to controlling costs. For example Bartlett (1991) suggests that the complexity of contracts required to control the supply of medical services through the market is such as to favour more traditional peer or "moral" control in the NHS. However in the eyes of liberal radical economists the gains to be made through the more effective provision of services in "quasi-markets", or in the "spinning-off" of activities formerly provided in-house, can be seen as more than off-setting the increase in transaction costs sustained by the community (Enthoven: 1985). An additional, but often unstated, benefit might be seen as deriving from the loss of collective bargaining leverage among long-term employees and the creation of a large pool of itinerant labour available for a "swarm" of "self-empowering" sub contractors bidding for spin-off services.

NPM IN THE NHS

The application of the NPM in the NHS can be seen to emphasize several unique aspects of service delivery in this sector. Among them the first must be that of testing the strategic dependence of managers on the expertise of the medical clinician in the delivery of care to the consumer. (The social institutionalisation of medicine considerably predates the application of Scientific Management.) Secondly the bottom-up emergence of medical care in Britain together with the artisanal nature of training and induction into the profession have combined to produce an enormous heterogeneity in local cultural norms and fractionation and conflict between procedural forms. A third concern of more recent origin is the Paretan distribution of resources toward what Vann-Wye (1992) describes as the individualistic-curative hospital-based methodologies rather than to communical-preventative modes of care.

The restructuring of formal authority within the NHS that followed the Griffiths proposals (1983) gave ultimate responsibility for the Service's functioning to general managers at all levels of service provision. The devolution of operational budgets to clinical departments accorded with an artisanal "firm" tradition within hospital management whilst imposing new hierarchical accountability on operational management drawn from the medical professions. It was, however, the 1991 introduction of a quasi-market relationship between providers of services and purchasers that created a new impetus towards the introduction of effective management. The rationale for reform was clearly based on that of providing choice to consumers through which suppliers would be pressurized into undertaking the sought-after efficient standardisation of their operations. One of the most significant elements in the creation of the internal market has been the role attributed to General Practitioners (GPs). As purchasers of services from directly managed units and self governing trusts they retain their time-honoured role as the professional agent of the individual consumer i.e. their patient.

THE ROLE OF THE GP

Since the passing of the 1911 Social Insurance Act the provision of primary care in the community has grown both as a function of (i) the growing numbers of GPs financed from publicly administered funds and (ii) from the quite separate provisions provided by Local (city and rural) Authorities (LAs). This differentiation and fragmentation of primary care provision was enshrined in the National Health Services Act of 1946 in spite of calls for a more integrated form of multi-purpose district modelled on that provided by some Labour run LAs in the 1930s. In part this decision seems to have reflected the Minister's own preferences but it is generally regarded as the outcome of a long drawn out negotiation with institutionalised interests (Bevan: 1976). (Similar Governmental compromises with professional interests over that period are to be seen in respect of the statutory provision of legal and public education and sundry other direct services.)

The subsequent evolution of the role of the GP within the NHS has been traced by Bryden (1992) who is inclined to an optimistic view of the manner in which the lynch-pin function accorded to GP sub-contractors will be accepted within the profession. From the narrow contractual position adopted by the GP at the start of the Service in 1948 practice management has grown to acquire the potential to become a base for "a consensus-managed primary health care team" (Bryden: 1992: 67).

By contrast Bartlett's (1991) entirely theoretical analysis throws doubt on the ability of purchasers (fund-holding GPs and Family Health Service Authorities [FHSAs]) to negotiate in a manner that will bring about an efficient transfer price for hospital services. Using a transaction cost perspective (TC) Bartlett suggests that, given the open ended nature of block contracts and the lack of a satisfactory basis for cost accounting, hospital providers will be forced into opportunistic behaviour vis-a-vis GP purchasers. Cost over-runs may be dispersed in new pricing decisions across the range of hospital provision or in the distribution of payments on Government equities but most of the risk will be passed to GP purchasers.

In order to guard against such supplier opportunism mechanisms have been created by the Act to monitor the performance of provider units through medical audit and through externally set performance targets. These mechanisms are seen by Bartlett as ensuring the continuation of high overhead costs of hierarchical limits to market exchanges. "Estimates of the number of additional accountants required to cope with the implementation of the internal market vary from 250 (Audit Commission) up to 1000 at a cost of œ25m". (Bartlett: 1991: 14). To this inner core of managerial capability has to be added the ever-growing periphery of "self-empowering" management consultants and trainers employed by both providers and users in the NHS or their largest suppliers, the drug companies (Malek *et al*: 1992).

General practitioners might argue otherwise with Barlett's attribution of motive for the role of medical audit. Indeed, it could be said that analysts of the NPM did not pay sufficient attention to the changing value system of professionals themselves. Whilst organisationally, the NHS has caused GPs to act as independent practitioners paid by item of service their professional training and culturally adopted value systems has tended towards paternalism. That such traditional paternalism may now be changing to a value system based on autonomy has been explored by Jensen and Mooney. They ask what is the effect of these changing value systems upon health policy and importantly "who holds the properly rights over which decision?" (Jensen and Mooney, 1990: 14). If indeed there has been a distinct change from paternalism to autonomy amongst individual doctors, (and this area does not appear to be extensively researched) then the collective value system still appears to be one of paternalism, in which case medical audit plays an important role in maintaining peer review and collective expertise.

FROM ARTISAN TO OPERATIONAL MANAGER?

In many respects the terms and conditions of service adopted for GPs in the 1946 Act most closely resembled those of the traditional artisanal piece-worker. Even after the inclusion of reimbursement for the costs of ancillary staff and premises in the late 1960s the managerial role formally accorded to GPs within the NHS was relatively small. Relationships with the wider hierarchy often seemed focused more on the central Doctors and Dentists (Pay) Review Body than on representation on local medical committees advising Executive Councils (now FHSAs). In the sense implied by institutional economists GPs were from the start players in a highly fractionated "internal market" in which piece-work prices provided a strong underlying link with the hierarchy.

Their physical and social isolation from peers severely diluted any collective identity. The pragmatic nature of their pastoral care inhibited the establishment of a knowledge-based discipline. The nature of the continued training and induction of GPs by attachment to hospital-based specialisms continues to reinforce a perceived reliance on these acute knowledge bases within medicine. Only in 1952 was the British College of General Practitioners established and mandatory training not established until thirty years later. The "Charter for the Family Doctor Service" produced by the British Medical Association's General Medical Services Committee in 1965 is seen by Bryden (op cit) as providing a basis for a new focus of identity within the profession. Since then both strategic management in the NHS and new recruits to community medicine have undergone a slow conversion to acceptance of a team management role for GPs.

In analysing trends in primary care over the last decade one might perhaps put a more realistic emphasis on the shift in Governmental emphasis towards "care in the community" as a result of economic pressures to constrain individualistic curative (hospital-based) methodologies in favour of less costly health-maintenance programmes. From public reportage there appears to be considerable scepticism among GPs towards the modes of illness-prevention currently favoured by NHS allocation of piece rates. In the reorganisation of practices towards a multi-purpose function and the attendant emergence of the new occupational status of practice-management financial inducements continue to provide the principal modes of "arms-length" strategic management.

In many respects, then, the operation of an internal market for the artisanal provision of care in the community has shaped a practitioner conception of competences based on the achievement of tangible concrete tasks easily recognisable by NHS administrators. The style of service delivery has been largely ignored. Broader goals such as the mapping of patient needs or epidemiological research has been elevated to staff functions within RHAs in a typically Tayloristic fashion.

GP's lack enthusiasm for collective responses to these mechanistic control structures. By the same token collective action of an altruistic nature is also rare. This is nowhere better illustrated than in the take-up for new forms of IT and diagnostic equipment. It may be argued that without suitable supporting infrastructures such individual investments have been of potentially limited value. It is, however, notable that two private agencies have discovered an enormously profitable value-added niche in the provision of "no cost option" computer systems to practices in exchange for aggregated patient information (Ferguson: 1991). The existence of this profitable bridge between suppliers and providers may be seen as symptomatic of the narrowly calculative nature of existing links between primary carers and other parts of the NHS and the inability of service managers to create and support rich information flows between the two levels of carers.

It is possible to interpret the form of internal market created in 1948 as having supported and reinforced the concept of the family doctor whose skills and knowledge base is of a highly idiosyncratic and tacit nature. As might be predicted by a TC analyst the history of primary care management has involved ever more complexity in provisions for contingent eventualities. In the context of current reforms the pivotal role assigned to GPs entails transactions creating boundaries to responsibilities and remunerations at a new level of complexity. For some practitioners an alternative of salaried status already appears as a more attractive option (Griffin: 1992).

At the other extreme, practitioners such as Bryden envisage that the GP (normally taken to be a fund-holder) will internalise transactions between the differentiated providers of community care by establishing a co-ordinative node between local networks within their organisations. Thus as a boundary spanning agent, the local practice will be seen as leading bottom-up innovation in primary care. The establishment of such nodal practices by a minority of GPs under conditions existing before the 1990 Act is taken as evidence of the viability of this model.

For the majority of GPs their strategic perspective appears still to be shaped by the vertical dependency of their practice on NHS stake-holders at different levels of hierarchical sanctioning. Shifting their frame of reference to encompass the strategic significance of horizontal alliances with a diverse set of other primary carers might well require proximal inducements of a kind that have not historically been present in the local context. Yet, movement away from reliance upon concrete proximal performance targets, typical of past and present sanctions, to a more conceptive overview of the system in which they are to play such a pivotal role might be considered to require feedback of a more intelligent nature. GPs have not lacked inter-group media. Over the past quarter century the number of tabloid newspapers financed by drug advertisers has multiplied faster than learned journals. Neither provide the type of performance data that has been produced in ad hoc research studies such as those of the Warwickshire Practice Feedback Study (Szczepura *et al*: 1992). Clearly the systemic adoption of such intelligently created data is long overdue.

Paradoxically, the GPs' claim to leadership in the provision of primary care is based on possession of a superior body of specialist knowledge. As in other areas of NPM the State's attempt to co-opt the professional worker into accountability for cost management, demands that his or her substantive task skills should be supplemented by those of the administrative manager. Team leadership is likely to require ability to use both administrative and social relational techniques. Nevertheless the GP's claim to authority originated from the structural basis of his or her esoteric expertise (Smith and Peterson: 1988). Present changes taking place both in the internal division of labour within the practice and in the re-establishment of inter-organisational boundaries are likely to feed back into modes of educating and inducting GPs, as well as adding burgeoning layers of post-graduate refresher courses. There is however a limit to the extension of these processes of professional qualification and choices will have to be made between specialised foci.

The present movement among a minority of practices to specialise in particular forms of treatment, particularly in minor surgery, might be seen as symptomatic of an eventual cross-practice division of labour (Wiggins: 1992). In this case the current adoption of purchaser-provider consortia by some practices might extend to a more substantive collaboration in the exchange of clients across the provision of specialised services. Should this evolution in the practice of communal medicine take place it is likely to impact on the career development of professionals and, perhaps, also on the emergence of new user-provider relations with secondary care.

Indeed, one of the consequences of the NHS reforms has been the re-evaluation of appropriate settings for acute medical care. Marks has been able to demonstrate both the theoretical and practical application of a "hospital at home" service (Marks 1991) where the key professional workers on a domiciliary scale will be general practitioners and specialised district nurses.

The consequences of such domiciliary based acute care are profound in their effect upon secondary care. It would mean a redefinition of the meaning of primary care beyond that of a diagnostic and therapeutic gatekeeping service, to possibly the key functional planning unit for health policy as opposed to the district general hospital. Work is in its early stages in S.E. Thames RHA to follow on from Marks's findings and to model the effects of new provisions such as extended GP practices possibly along a polyclinic model and GP staffed community hospitals with an extended role.

To the client (i.e. patient or "lay-person") social relations between primary carers and hospital-based specialists often appear tenuous and extremely distant. (Ritualistic exchanges of letters seems to prevent even the adoption of fax in referrals!) Such relations contrast with many supplier-user relations in industry through which user innovations are often conveyed back up the supply chain. The relative isolation of hospital-based invention from the 90% of care provided by GPs might appear to be significant obstacle to medical innovation (Shaw: 1992).

FHSAS PRODUCT CHAMPIONS OR NEW BUREAUCRATS?

The role of local area regulators has been extended and reinforced by the 1990 Act. As well as being responsible for co-ordinating funding bids and for their allocation, FHSAs and DHAs have become responsible for interpreting and monitoring performance standards set by their own strategies as well as those set by RHAs under the NHS Executive. Up to now two distinctive thrusts in their activities can be observed.

One is that of clarifying the rules and data upon which choices and contests are to be allowed within the internal market. In this activity they act on remit from the RHA and National Executive as they do in the collection and primary analysis of performance data. They have also a responsibility for the allocation of funds based on preliminary and, necessarily crude assessments of need. (The "claw-back" of funds from practices that under spent their estimated budgets in the first year of operation under the new rules, demonstrated the extent to which practice managers continued their attempt to maximise private returns on cost savings.)

In the setting of standards there has evidently been considerable co-operation across providers and purchasers at the district level. In this sense Bartlett's fear of the high overhead costs involved in the clarification of market signals over a long time frame may have been avoided by the negotiation of conventional norms within a bureaucratic arena. However the question that underlies a great deal of GP opinion formation at present is the extent to which this collaboration in the regulation of the internal market will result in a progressive erosion of GP choices in regard to both the purchase of hospital services and the governance of fund-holding practices.

This is a fear that might be seen as being reinforced by the appointment of locality managers by some FHSAs designed to facilitate and co-ordinate practice management towards the achievement of nationally set performance targets. The historically fragmented organisation of general practice might be seen to demand this type of facilitating agency if progress is to be made by FHSA General Management towards the achievement of their hierarchically set targets. Yet the very individualism that brought about this fragmentation, and which continues to attract the current generation of GPs into primary care, is seen to be placed at risk by the imposition of structured co-ordination. Small wonder then that a suspicion of "creaming" of GP allowances by RHAs and FHSAs has been voiced and that demands for a more transparent allocative system have followed the first year of operations (Griffin 1992 *op cit*).

The second major thrust in the strategy of some FHSAs has been that of orchestrating the creation of multi-purpose care management at practice level along the lines described by Bryden (1992). Responding to the short term need to rationalise long-term hospital facilities the South East Thames RHA has encouraged FHSAs within its jurisdiction to promote "one-stop health shops" in which specialist consultants will outwork in the diagnosis and treatment of acute illness (Cooper: 1992). Within the same region the East Sussex FHSA has established a number of pilot projects in the care management of elderly and disabled clients. These bring together all locally provided services at practice level (Royston and Hoddinott: 1991).

For these initiatives to diffuse beyond the level of pilot projects demands an impetus that has not been found in the innumerable "demonstrator projects" financed within the NHS over nearly half a century. Managers of FHSAs are strategically well placed to intervene in the creation of new boundaries to the provision of primary care along lines that represent functionally effective groupings of carers rather than vested interest. They are sufficiently close to the operational needs of client groups to be able to distinguish the resources required in their satisfaction. Equally they are in the position to recognise and show sensitivity to the bases upon which practitioner interests become vested in particular proprietorial rights. In the process of the re negotiating, boundaries between interests they are better placed than national or regional executives to establish locally relevant trade-offs and to bring about a movement of interest through the creation of mutually beneficial (variable-sum) outcomes from cross boundary collaboration (Teram: 1991).

A real opportunity for the strategic role of the FHSA's to be asserted could come about with the 1993 implementation of community care legislation, following on from "Caring for People" 1989. As joint planners of primary and community care provision FHSAs are already required to contribute to the joint strategic plans between DHAs, Local Authority Social Services and local voluntary organisations for the Annual Joint Care Plans some of the more advanced purchasing consortia are now approaching a more, informed joint purchasing of services, where FHSAs and DHAs and some social service agencies have joint contracts to purchase. (SELCA - South East London Community Authority, Bromley Health and Dudley). The general practitioner may well believe that such top down planning will result in a new multi-disciplinary questioning of their professional authority. The essence of community care in the case management approach, which is dependent upon key workers or a team based approach of which the general practitioner is only one member. A future strategy of the FHSAs may well be to become central to a new organisation similar to the US group of community oriented primary carers (COPC). Weiner and Ferris, use this example to show how the disciplines of primary and community care can be merged with the discipline of epidemiology (Weiner and Ferris, 1990)

In the longer term, the role of executives within the NHS structure might itself become subjected to radical change. Over the history of the Service organisation change has been generally regarded as a "top down" process (Pettigrew *et al* 1992). The creation of relatively autonomous and operationally responsible groups of carers might be expected to give rise to "bottom-up" pressures for innovation on a scale and in areas not previously regarded as dynamic. Most inventions in the NHS have been confined to clinical diagnosis and treatment in hospitals in which the UK is still internationally famous. For the current reforms to be seen as successful they should give use to similar achievements in primary care delivery. There is, however, unlikely ever to be the same level of private (manufacturer-donated) sponsorship or reward of public standing that is presently attached to radical innovations in the curing of acute illness. The need for internal sponsorship for communal innovation is therefore all the more important.

Key activities / Levels	CORE PROCESSES		OVERLYING PROCESSES	
	Definition	**Impetus**	**Strategic context**	**Structural context**
Corporate Management (RHA/NHS)	Monitoring	Authorising	Rationalising	Structuring
	Organisational Championship			*Selecting*
New Ventures Management (FHSA)	Coaching, Stewardship	Strategic building	Delineating	Negotiating
	Product Championship			
Practice leader/ venture manager	Technical & need linking	Strategic forcing	Gatekeeping idea Generating Bootlegging	Questioning

Figure 1. The Stepped Process of Botton-Up Innovating
(based on Burgelman and Sayles: 1988)

The process by which the internal contest for support is conducted within one large American corporation is illustrated in Figure 1 below, which is based on the work of Burgelman and Sayles (1988). It is one which assumes the same fractional struggle for recognition among operational groups as that existing in the NHS. (This is often seen as a characteristic of Anglo—Saxon culturally-determined predispositions!) It requires that in order to achieve recognition at each level of the organisation an invention has to be sponsored by a key individual and translated into terms that are meaningful within the higher order of strategic significance. It demands also that managing executives should be constantly scanning their bureaucratically prescribed domains for competing examples of creation rather than regulating for conformity. At the same time the setting of strategic directions also means willing the means to their achievement. For example the take up of computers in general practice has been reported as being in decline even though it has not reached the level achieved in other service sectors (Barrowcliffe: 1991). Until the national infrastructure exists for the deployment of IT to its full potential in the control of disease as well as for local "bean counting" exercises it is unlikely that local initiatives will be seen as significant or lead to professionally based emulation. (Ahmad: 1992)

CONCLUSIONS

The fears expressed by academic critics of NPM had largely to do with the stress laid on the achievement of short term financial targets focused on achieving economy and efficiency. Complementing these misgivings have been suggestions that such short-term pressures will undermine trust within peer-group "clans". These informal mechanisms as seen to have worked in a way that ensured the honesty and integrity of the system of governance within the public sector (Hood: 1991).

By contrast, radical economists saw such relationships as institutionalised blockages to the achievement of effective service delivery. Only by extending market forces so that they operated within and between operational units in sectors such as higher education and health, could one ensure that co-ordinative linkages brought about an effective delivery of services required and selected by consumers.

In this paper we have observed a few of the early responses among GPs to the quasi-market being constructed within the NHS by the 1990 Act. It has been suggested that the primary care provided by GPs has always been shaped by a sub-contracting relationship within an internal market. In reality the present changes are most fruitfully interpreted as creating new demands upon primary carers in the reconceptualisation of the strategic context of their role.

In the learning process that NHS management have to undertake, FHSAs have to perform the dual role of clarifying the immediate operational and pricing procedures by which market contests will be regulated while also acting as the primary orchestrator of change at community level. It is in the significance attached to the latter role by FHSA management, and by those above them whose responsibility it is to provide a national infrastructure, that NPM in primary care will have to be judged.

If, the desire to re-establish clear operating norms, leads to an assumption of greater reliance on hierarchical authority by RHAs and FHSA then it seems likely that their emphasis in NPM will be upon the adoption of Scientific Management of a kind that has helped to bring about the decline of private industry in the UK. If on the other hand, the desire for clarity in procedural forms is tempered by a realisation of the need to create conditions necessary for cross-functional collaboration in service delivery — at the point of delivery — then a different emphasis in strategic implementation could emerge.

This emphasis might itself be born out of the needs of short-term crisis, as in the case of SE Thames RHA. It will, however, be nurtured by a desire to sponsor and to recognise internal initiative in a manner inimical to the mechanistic application of Scientific Management techniques. In the face of long-established vested interests, with deep roots in the social values of wider society, it might seem managerially sound to take the long view in both the establishment of procedural parameters within the NHS and in the more important task of shifting professional frames of reference.

REFERENCES

Ahmad S (1992) "Innovation and the Politics of Information Systems" in R. Loveridge and K. Starkey Continuity and Crisis in the NHS - the politics of design and innovation in health care, Buckingham: Open University Press.

Barrowcliffe M. (1991) "GP Computer use is in decline" GP 8 November: 100.

Bartlett W. (1991) "Quasi-Markets and Contracts: a markets and hierarchies perspective on NHS reform" Studies in Decentralisation and Quasi-Markets No. 3   School of Advanced Urban Studies Bristol: University of Bristol.

Bevan A. (1976) In Place of Fear, Wakefield: EP Publishing.

Bovaird T., Gregory D. and Martin S., (1991) "Improved Performance in Local Economic Development: a warm embrace or an artful sidestep?" Public Administration, 69, Spring, 103-119.

Bryden P. (1992) "The Future of Primary Care" in R. Loveridge and K. Starkey (eds) Continuity and Crisis in the NHS - the politics of design and innovation in Health Care, Buckingham: Open University Press.

Burgelman R.A. and Sayles L.R. (1988) Inside Corporate Innovation - strategy, structure and Managerial Skills, New York: Free Press.

Child J. and Loveridge R. (1990) Information Technology in European Services, Oxford: Basil Blackwell.

Cooper C. (1992) "GPs open doors for one-stop health shop", Doctor, 10 December, 27.

Dertouzos M. Lester R.K., Solow R. (1989: 1990 end) Made in America, New York: Harper.

Enthoven A. (1985) Reflections on the Management of the National Health Service, London: Nuffield Provincial Hospital Trust.

Ferguson A. (1991) "On the Fast Track to success in the 1990s", Business on Sunday, Independent, 28 April, 12.

Griffin M (1992) "How FHSA fund transfers may prove costly for GPs", Money Pulse 22 June 1.

Hood C. (1990) "Beyond the public bureaucracy state? Public Administration in the 1990s" London School of Economic Inaugural Lecture, 16 January.

Hood C (1991) "A Public Management for all Seasons", Public Administration, 69, Spring 3-19.

Malek M.H., Davey P.G. and Scott W. (1992) "Professionals as Gatekeepers: the role of doctors in the pharmaceutical value chain" in R. Loveridge and K. Starkey (eds) Continuity and Crisis in the NHS - the politics of design and innovation in Health Care, Buckingham: Open University Press.

Pettigrew A., Ferlie E., and McKee L. (1992) Shaping Strategic Change: making change in large organizations, London: Sage.

Pirie M. (1988) Privatisation, Aldershot: Wildwood House.

Pollitt C. Harrison S., Hunter D.J. and Marroch G. (1991) "General Management in the NHS: the initial impact, 1983-1988", Public Administration, 69, Spring, 61-83.

Rhodes R.A.W. (ed) (1991) "The New Public Management", Public Administration, 69.1.

Royson S. and Hoddinott D. (1991) "Care Management: working with GPs in East Sussex" in Caring for People, 3 January 1.

Shaw B (1992) "The Diffusion of Innovation in Clinical Equipment" in R. Loveridge and K. Starkey (eds) op cit Continuity and Crisis in the NHS - the politics of design and innovation in Health Care, Buckingham: Open University Press.

Smith P.B. and Peterson M.F. (1988) Leadership, Organizations and Culture, London, Sage.

Szczepura A., Wilmot J., Davies C. (1992) "Better Information, Better Primary Care?" The Warwickshire Practice Feedback Study, Coventry: Health Services Research Unit, Warwick Business School Research Bureau, University of Warwick.

Teram E (1991) Interdisciplinary Teams and Control of Clients: a socio-technical perspective", Human Relations, 44, 4, 343-356.

Toom S. (1991) "Salaried Service Re-think" Pulse 26 October 7.

Vann-Wye G (1992) "Hospitals in the UK: a history of Design-Innovation" in R. Loveridge and K. Starkey (eds) op cit Continuity and Crisis in the NHS - the politics of design and innovation in Health Care, Buckingham: Open University Press.

Wiggins B (1922) "The Cutting edge of General Practice" Financial Pulse, 10 March 54-58.

4 Strategic Information Systems Planning for Primary Care Prescribing

BRIAN FROST & JOHN SILLINCE

Sheffield University Management School

THE NEED FOR STRATEGIC INFORMATION SYSTEMS PLANNING

Integrating Information Management (IM) with organisational strategy is the next great challenge for the National Health Service (NHS). The publication of the *Health of the Nation* white paper (DoH 1991a, 1992a) committed the government to a crucial change of direction in the NHS. Information Management and Technology (IM&T) has a fundamental role to play in this process of change. In its first 45 years the health service has arguably been driven more by providers than by purchasers: a veneer of central planning has been superimposed on a random collection of beds and doctors. In fact, until recently, IM&T has almost been invisible in the Health Service. The two main exceptions were the Family Health Service Authorities (FHSAs) and the Prescription Prescribing Authority (PPA). The former were obliged to automate their patient registers and the latter had to automate prescription pricing. Strategic information systems planning (SISP) is necessary in order to maximise the effectiveness of information resources. By SISP is meant the planning of Information Systems (IS) for organisational benefit using a systematic methodology. In the absence of SISP, information resources will not support strategic planning within the NHS.

Todays health service strategy is consciously articulated by ministers and the Health Service Management Executive interprets these statements and communicates them to the rest of the Health Service. The top-level NHS goals are currently threefold: first, to maintain and improve the health of population; second, to provide a quality service to individuals; and third, to deploy available resources effectively and efficiently (Malone-Lee 1992). In practice, the implementation of these goals will be mediated through a number of Commissioners (DoH 1992f) who will be based in existing health authorities, such as Regional Health Authorities (RHAs), District Health Authorities (DHAs) and FHSAs. Formerly, these same authorities

Managerial Issues in the Reformed NHS. Edited by M.Malek, P.Vacani, J.Rasquinha & P.Davey
© 1993 John Wiley & Sons Ltd

planned levels of provision and dealt directly or indirectly with providers. Today, as Commissioners, these authorities will want to maximise health gain for their resident populations. Their concerns will include some of the following: targeting particular needs; finding effective means of satisfying these needs; promoting good health within the local population; and finding effective means of caring for and treating the sick. The intention is that the Commissioners, rather than the providers, will now be in the driving seat. To some extent it can be said that bottom-up planning, based on providers' perception of need, is now to be replaced by top-down planning based on the Commissioners' assessment of health gain.

Information systems are clearly required to monitor the implementation of the overall strategy at both local and higher levels. At a minimum, IS will satisfy this requirement by providing both feedback on implementation of existing plans (such as detailed budgeting, variance analysis, ratio analysis, standard product costing) and information contributing to future initiatives in support of top-level NHS goals (such as planning interventions affecting the pattern of smoking, and, coronary related disease). In addition, Commissioners will also need IS with the following capabilities: monitoring and managing contracts; exercising financial control; linking individual records within and between health service organisations; preserving confidentiality; tracking population movements; and providing a basic register of their resident population. These features are closely related to the critical success factors discussed below.

The overall strategy of the Health Service needs to be interpreted in terms of its component sub-systems such as the primary and secondary health care sectors. Each sub-system has to make an appropriate contribution to the NHS value chain and IM can assist in controlling the use of resources, providing a balanced IS portfolio and enhancing linkages between value-creating activities. The focus of this paper is on the primary care sector and in particular on primary care prescribing. Politically, the importance of primary care prescribing was recognised with the publication of *Improving Prescribing* (DoH 1990a). The changeover to fundholding by GPs will further enhance their role. More recently, the Secretary of State for Health has said: 'GPs and their teams have a vital role in helping us to meet targets and improve the health of the nation' (Bottomley 1992).

SISP WITHIN THE NHS

NHS IS developments can be viewed as a portfolio, and both current and future IS portfolios have strategic significance. The situation is unusually complicated within the NHS. Not only is it necessary to make the conventional distinction between the organisation as a whole and its strategic business units, but there is also a growing awareness that a market-based system may develop as more hospitals and GP practices adopt trust and fundholding status respectively, and Commissioners become separated from providers. The current IS portfolio must reflect the NHS as it is today, although future developments may make the concept of a single NHS portfolio less meaningful.

The NHS is an organisation whose constituent parts have similar problems requiring compatible solutions. Some experiments must be encouraged and monitored, while others ought to be avoided. Information and results should be publicised, and specialist advice disseminated. IT infrastructure also needs to conform to certain organisational standards. For these reasons, some element of central direction of NHS IS development is justified and NHS IS can be viewed strategically as forming a portfolio comprising distinct types of IS development (Earl, 1989):

- *Early successes* providing high payoffs in the short term earn credibility with top management, while making a useful addition to the portfolio. By way of example, PACTLINE (supporting the Indicative Prescribing Scheme by providing access for FHSA Medical Advisers to certain categories of PACT reports) may be regarded as falling into this category. The development of micro-packages such as the recently released GP practice profiles by the FHSA Computer Unit in Exeter is another example.

- *Glittering prizes* providing high payoffs sometime in the long term include applications with strategic significance leading to eventual competitive advantage. Development, however, is risky enough to deter most competitors from investment. An example here might be Decision Support Systems for GPs harnessing expert systems' technology by offering GPs some of the knowledge and experience (in software form) of consultants.

- *Sweetmeats* are systems offering low payoffs in the short term. Their advantage is that development time is short (usually less than a year) and their delivery on time is almost assured. A succession of sweetmeats offers users a continual enhancement in service. Examples include planned upgrades (or rewrites) of PACTLINE, and GP-FHSA Links. Action in-hand following *Working for Patients* (DoH 1989) such as 'cleaning-up' FHSA Registers with respect to NHS numbers and post-codes also fall into this category.

- *Back burners* offering low, uncertain payoffs sometime in the long term should be postponed until their future prospects are more assured. Examples in this category might include patient-held records on 'smart cards'.

- *Failures* happen in all portfolios and are unavoidable. For example, the Regional Information Systems Plan ran from 1982 to 1990, when it was abandoned.

Promoting Better Health and *Working for Patients* (DoH 1887 1989) changed the role and responsibilities of FHSAs (formerly Family Practitioner Committees). The IS developments promised as a result of these publications (see Appendix 1) provide further examples of IS developments mainly falling into the Sweetmeats category.

CENTRALISATION VERSUS DECENTRALISATION OF IS DEVELOPMENT

The NHS has, for many years, exhibited some of the features of a centrally-planned system with its familiar tension between centralising and decentralising forces. The one billion pound IS investment in the NHS is made within a pluralist decision environment (BJHCC 1992a). This has encouraged competition amongst suppliers who have adapted to particular needs or special niches, and this in turn has encouraged a high degree of experimentation. The extent to which health agencies should be permitted to make their own decisions about IS development, rather than adhering to some centrally devised plan, is subject to debate. One view, expressed at a recent conference, is that 'Chief executives and financial directors are often not willing to let management (functions) go to the users' (BJHCC 1991).

There is evidence of over-direction from the top. As yet strategic planning of IT for primary care is not well developed and there is evidence that the computerisation of primary care was rushed to fit in with the political timetable set by fundholding changes (Sillince 1992). Also, clinical directors are being encouraged to purchase expensive case-mix management systems before they have fully worked out requirements.

Central direction, however, does have some advantages. For example, the development of standards, minimum data sets, common codes for all clinical areas, and classification systems have to be managed centrally. A GP practice's transition to fundholder status depends partly on computer sophistication, again a centrally-made judgement. Likewise a hospital's transition to trust status is judged partly on a hospital's IT infrastructure. Recently, a health agency in the south of England had to admit to mistaken procurement decisions (BJHCC 1992b), and these mistakes might have been avoided had there been more central direction.

Decentralisation can be particularly useful when it leads to vigorous experimentation. Some of these experiments are noted below, and a number of them have interesting implications for information transfer between the primary and secondary sectors. The appropriate degree of centralisation (or decentralisation) affecting primary care and its IM&T developments are summarised in Table 1. This table is influenced by McFarlan (1983), Tricker (1982), and Feeny (1987).

In a commercial organisation an IT Steering Committee frequently decides on priorities and other matters relating to the IS portfolio. Such a group did not exist in the NHS until recently, when the NHS Management Executive established the Information Management Group, which last year published the *Handbook for IM&T Specialists* (DoH 1992g). Essentially, an overall national strategy has been drafted for the next ten years. The theme of which is that a 'national lead' will be followed by 'local implementation'. Where it is unclear what the national lead should be, local projects will be established and monitored. Some of these experiments are listed in an Appendix to the *Handbook*.

Table 1. Centralising versus decentralising forces in IT development

Strategic action	Towards centralisation	Towards decentralisation
Direction	Adjusting funding incentives to induce GPs to invest in IT	Removing bureaucratic controls particularly from fundholders
	Ensure fundholders make savings	Enable fundholders to have 'whip hand' over providers
	Direct savings towards approved projects	Promote competition amongst IT suppliers
	Monitor problems between GPs and IT suppliers	Encourage diversity in fundholders' IS
	Promote and police standards on NHS numbers, Read Codes, administrative registers, etc.	Enable GPs to become less dependent on NHS hierarchy
Development	Promote GP access to patient information regardless of location	Permit patients to access their records
	Create attractive career opportunities for IT staff	Reassure patients about security
	Ensure compatible communication and local network standards	Break down barriers between end users and IT specialists
Operations	Benefit from economies of scale, particularly in EDI	Promote GP's ownership of data (and thereby ensure high data quality)
	Ensure availability of prescribing data to Medical Advisers and FHSA	Promote GP as primary care expert
	Ensure integration of data from diverse sources	Encourage GP computing

The corporate attitude to technological risk requires discussion. It is widely agreed that patient information should be kept 'secure' and 'confidential' (DoH 1992g). What is the risk of loss of confidentiality of patient clinical data? What are the safeguards against unauthorised data access? What contingency plans exist for when systems break down? How are these risks evaluated? These questions are not peculiar to the NHS, but the personal nature of the data makes action more imperative. Legal issues also require careful attention. For example, the status of documents such as contracts is still difficult to assess in the eventual context of electronic data interchange within the NHS.

The IM&T strategy requires continuous review particularly in respect to training and information dissemination. The move to fundholder status is largely dependent upon the growth of computer awareness. IT awareness poses different and perhaps larger problems for GPs and their small teams than for doctors and other professionals working on large sites.

Organisations are known to pass through different IT stages: from a few IT pioneers; to rapid uncontrolled experimentation; to central over-direction; to decentralisation together with an integrated cost control system. Until recently the NHS IT function was over-centralised. In IT terms the NHS is not a mature organisation. Considerable gains can be made from cost control and a reduction in paperwork in nearly every part of the NHS including GP practices (allegedly £0.25 million per year in one GP practice). For the foreseeable future properly managed IT investment will be cost-effective.

PRIMARY CARE PRESCRIBING AS A STRATEGIC BUSINESS UNIT

Most patients make contact with the NHS via the primary care sector. This sector produces a related group of services fulfilling the normal criteria for a strategic business unit. Responsibility centres include FHSAs, NHS pharmacy and appliance contractors, and GP practices, all of which have traditional roles. The GP practice acted as a gatekeeper to high technology care (such as hospital services), and, if high technology care was not required, the GP's alternative role was that of low-cost caring typically discharged by prescribing drugs. Pharmacy and appliance contractors dispensed most GP prescriptions, and FHSAs covered routine administrative chores such as NHS prescription and practice capitation payments.

In the past the NHS treated each responsibility centre as a discretionary expense centre. Following the introduction of the Indicative Prescribing Scheme (IPS) in April 1991, GP practices and FHSAs are increasingly viewed as non-discretionary expense centres whose budgets are to be estimated beforehand and are subsequently used to assess efficiency of operations (DoH 1990). At regional level the average percentage overspend for 1991/92 was 8.2 per cent (Hepburn 1992). The 1991/92 IPS budgets (Indicative Prescribing Amounts or IPAs) were set too low - the two-year uplift was subsequently assessed at 18.5 per cent. In fact the increase (in Net Ingredient Cost) of 12 per cent over the previous year is attributable to a number of factors: health promotion and screening resulting in more drugs being prescribed; the transfer of prescribing responsibility from hospital consultants to GPs; increased patient demand; and increased activity from pharmaceutical company representatives (Hepburn 1992).

It is widely believed that some wasteful GP prescribing still exists: adherents quote the observed variation between individual GPs or practices. There are a number of questions which affect primary care prescribing. Can GPs avoid wasteful prescribing? Can generic prescribing continue to increase? Will FHSAs be able to keep within budget in future? Will forecasting of IPAs become more accurate (Hepburn 1992)?

Fundholding GPs also raise some interesting issues because potentially they control high-technology purchasing. It is expected that fundholders will demand more choice and higher quality for their patients. From April 1993 1 in 4 of the population will be cared for by fundholders. IT in the past had little or no importance for most GPs: inevitably, the future importance of IT will increase greatly for all responsibility centres in primary care. In terms of the strategic grid, IT will move from support to strategic categories (McFarlan 1983).

A PROPOSED IS PLANNING FRAMEWORK

The three aspects of our proposed planning framework are intended to reflect three strategic concerns of management:

Top down clarification

The formulation of business objectives is integral to *The Health of the Nation* both in its Green Paper (DoH 1991a) and White Paper (DoH 1992a) versions. The Department (DoH 1991b) suggested some ministerial priorities, and the NHS Management Executive interpreted these in more specific terms for Regional General Managers and Chairmen: see, for example, EL(91)70, (DoH 1991c), which was later updated by EL(92)47, (DoH 1992b). Also, the Department has published guidelines on business plans for the different levels of the NHS and methods of implementation (DoH 1992c) as well as examples of policy fulfilment (such as DoH 1992d).

Top level objectives such as those in DoH (1991a; 1991b; 1991c) have not been based upon any theoretical principles (Smith 1991). For example, economic efficiency has not been the driving force behind these statements. There is no attempt to specify and parameterise health inputs competing for scarce resources, and individual programmes do not win or lose resources based upon estimates of costs and benefits of their outputs (Mooney 1991). Instead the objectives focus on specific treatment groups and quality of service. It may be argued that the data does not yet exist for comparisons to be made based upon theoretical concerns (such as economic efficiency). The non-theoretical and arbitrary nature of past and current objectives, however, means that future moves towards them will become more difficult to justify. The pragmatic emphasis of current policy on performance evaluation is underlined by the narrow medical and NHS-focused definition of health implicit in government health strategy (Smith 1991), and the inclusion of no less than six evaluation criteria (that is, equity, efficiency, accessibility, appropriateness, effectiveness, and responsiveness) in some recent NHS Management Executive advice (DoH 1992b).

```
┌─────────────────────────────────────────────────────────────┐
│ Three top-level NHS goals are:                              │
│  •        to maintain and improve the health of population  │
│  •        to provide a quality service to individuals       │
│  •        to deploy available resources effectively and efficiently │
└─────────────────────────────────────────────────────────────┘
```

⇓

```
┌─────────────────────────────────────────────────────────────┐
│ NHS Management Executive objectives for primary care        │
│    prescribing are:                                          │
│  •        to monitor the operation of all GP IPAs           │
│  •        to monitor Regional non-cash limited FHSA drug budgets │
│  •        to encourage and support practices wishing to become │
│           fundholders                                        │
└─────────────────────────────────────────────────────────────┘
```

⇓

```
┌─────────────────────────────────────────────────────────────┐
│ Current policy implies the following critical success factors: │
│  •        keep GP prescribing expenditure within existing IPAs │
│  •        increase generic and rational prescribing         │
│  •        maintain up-to-date population registers for each FHSA │
│  •        guarantee confidentiality and security of individual records │
└─────────────────────────────────────────────────────────────┘
```

⇓

```
┌─────────────────────────────────────────────────────────────┐
│ Information requirements implicit in these objectives are:  │
│  •        feedback on implementation of existing IPAs e.g. detailed │
│           budgeting, variance analysis, ratio analysis      │
│  •        information contributing to setting realistic IPAs in future │
│  •        a basic register of each FHSA's resident population utilising │
│           practice records                                   │
│  •        information concerning rational prescribing       │
│  •        the ability to link individual records within and between │
│           health service organisations                       │
│  •        the confidentiality and security of individual patient records │
└─────────────────────────────────────────────────────────────┘
```

Figure 1. Information Requirements for Primary Care Prescribing
(the source for the Management Executive objectives is DoH 1991c)

The way in which the three top-level business goals, listed in the first section, impinge upon each strategic business unit and its information requirements needs to be understood. Some of the issues relevant to primary care prescribing are shown in figure 1 (DoH 1991c) and they are discussed below in more detail. The clarification of IS requirements generally implies top-down analysis and successive refinement moving from general to specific objectives in a quasi-deductive manner. Some work has already begun (for example,. DoH 1992b; 1992c). Figure 1 also shows some necessary elements of such a process.

Bottom up evaluation

Management needs to be informed on current IS applications. Existing IS may provide relevant pointers to achieving the desired portfolio. This evaluation is best approached 'bottom up' by means of fieldwork, surveys, and audits consulting GPs and other users and specialists in FHSAs and DHAs. It is necessarily judgmental, involving many (and possibly conflicting) clinical and administrative opinions. There are several non-technical questions which ought to be raised about existing IS. Does feedback from sources such as PACT alter GP behaviour, particularly in respect of IPAs? Is PACT and its associated systems sufficiently refined to detect changes in GP behaviour attributable to whether or not the practice has fundholding status? Unsolicited feedback of information may have little influence on GPs' behaviour (Hamley 1981), whereas peer group pressure or regular practice meetings may have beneficial effects (Pringle 1992). GPs may perhaps respond even better to impersonal information (such as from a decision-support system) which is available ex ante rather than ex post. Such systems might encourage GPs to participate readily in data collection rather than seeing it as an end in its own right (Sandiford 1992). Does PACT permit any inferences to be made about inappropriate prescribing? Should practice formularies become more common? Can existing IS such as PACT offer useful information to Medical Audit Advisory Groups?

Innovation

Innovation in NHS is frequently undertaken via local experiments or projects. There is a good reason for encouraging innovation through this particular route. The NHS is a large organisation and failures can prove expensive. Also, in the past and possibly still today, the principles of line management and organisational hierarchy have not gained acceptance at provider level. The relative status of two important professional groups (doctors and managers) was unclear or weighted in favour of doctors with clinical responsibility. Today the situation is complicated by the radical nature of recent reforms. Few can be completely certain of NHS organisational structure in ten years time. For this and similar reasons, locally-based experiments are being encouraged.

Some early examples are worth noting: the Exeter Care Card project (HMSO 1990) in which cards were used to allow patients access to their medical records, and to provide a mechanism for the movement of information between the different parts of the primary and secondary healthcare systems, and projects involving bar-code identity systems (Manser 1992; Wijay 1992). The *Developing IS for Purchasers Project* (DISP; DoH 1992f) provides a more focused IM&T example exploring contract management, health needs assessment, management information and population register and health related events. In fact four project sites are investigating different IS solutions to DISP. The intention is to use the experiences of these sites to stimulate interest elsewhere in the NHS.

CRITICAL SUCCESS FACTORS IN PRIMARY CARE PRESCRIBING

Critical success factors (CSFs) have gained acceptance as the cornerstone of a number of SISP methodologies. The CSFs specified in Figure. 1 are derived from the business objectives for primary care prescribing, and measures of operational efficiency, or managerial performance indicators, could in turn be derived from them.. The CSF approach is consistent with additional top-down decomposition and successive refinement by lower managers. One advantage of this approach is that it draws attention to information needs and so avoids an over-hasty commitment to specifying solutions.

The justification for the selection of critical success factors shown in Figure. 1 lies in current policy towards primary care prescribing. Neither *Improving Prescribing* nor the *Handbook* contain any references to CSFs. Hence a brief summary justifying our selection is given:

- Prescribing expenditure by GPs is to be kept within existing budgets (IPAs), otherwise practice drug expenditure could escalate unpredictably leading to an unwelcome increase in Regional non-cash limited FHSA drug budgets which would have to be met by the Treasury.
- Increases in generic and rational prescribing are widely thought to result in cost-savings without any adverse consequences for quality of care.
- Inter-practice variation in IPAs needs to be reduced. Such variation, after allowing for demographic differences such as age-sex variations, and possibly epidemiological differences, between practices, is taken as prima facie evidence that some prescriptions are unnecessary.
- Information flow should increase between practices, pharmacies, the PPA, and FHSAs. For example, there is no guarantee that FHSA patient registers are currently up-to-date. The source of this information lies with practices. Hence each FHSA can better monitor population movements if the GP-FHSA Links project leads to a quicker movement of data between practices and itself. Further developments in this area could benefit pharmacies and the PPA. Relevant population-based information is also required by other health agencies including Commissioners, and this particular CSF has planning implications going beyond the immediate needs of primary care prescribing. The Sheffield GP Links project is also laying down lines of communication between its GPs and local hospitals.
- A guarantee of confidentiality and security of individual records is thought to be a *sine qua non* for increased automation linking different health agencies

The general background against which these CSFs have to be judged is that IM&T strategy must favour both seamless patient care and the free communication of person-based information (DoH 1992g). More generally within primary care as a whole GPs need a freer flow of information in respect of morbidity patterns, investigations, hospital referrals, waiting times, bookings, and discharges.

ALIGNING IT INVESTMENT WITH BUSINESS NEEDS

The NHS Management Executive recognises the need for an IM&T strategy (DoH 1992g). The current statement of intentions suggests that five principles will guide future developments. Information will be person-based, derived from transaction or operational systems, avoiding data redundancy wherever possible and shared across NHS IS. An assurance is offered that information will only be made available to authorised users who need to know it. The importance of GPs is acknowledged. Practice management systems are to be enhanced by allowing GPs to make the best possible decisions regarding 'referring, prescribing and investigating' (DoH 1992g). GPs should have up-to-date information on healthcare received by their patients in other locations, for example, in an Accident and Emergency hospital department. The realisation of the 'vision' is expected to be facilitated by local projects and by developing a national infrastructure. Local strategies are expected to be guided by the national strategy and local needs.

SISP methodology attempts to ensure that IT makes a substantial contribution to achieving organisational and business goals. The visionary approach currently in favour needs to be controlled at least in its early stages. The NHS has not achieved the level of IM&T sophistication at which local implementation can reliably deliver the consistency and quality which the visionary approach deserves, either in primary care prescribing or in most other NHS business units.

REFERENCES

Bottomley, V. (1992), 'Primary care: the way forward', *Management in General Practice*, 6, 11.

BJHCC (1991), 'Management blamed for failure of IT projects', *British Journal of Health Care Computing*, April, 8-9.

BJHCC (1992a), 'NHS spends £1 billion a year on IT', *British Journal of Health Care Computing*, September, 4.

BJHCC (1992b), Editorial, *British Journal of Health Care Computing*, June, 4.

DoH (1987) *Promoting Better Health: the Government's Programme for Improving Primary Health Care*, Cm. 249, Department of Health, HMSO, London.

DoH (1989), *Working for Patients*, Cmnd. 555, HMSO, London.

DoH (1990a), *Improving Prescribing. The implementation of the GP Indicative Prescribing Scheme*, Department of Health, 1990.

DoH (1990b), *Working for Patients, Framework for Information Systems: The Next Steps*, Information Management Group, Department of Health, HMSO, London.

DoH (1990c), *Working for Patients, Framework for Information Systems: Overview,* Working Paper 11, Information Management Group, Department of Health, HMSO, London.

DoH (1991a), *The Health of the Nation: a summary of the Government's Proposals: a consultative document for health in England and Wales,* June, HMSO, London.

DoH (1991b), Secretary of State's Statement, Mission, Goals, Priorities, and Key Challenges, 1991/2 to 1994/5, Department of Health, London.

DoH (1991c), EL(91)70, NHS Management Executive goals and objectives 1991/2 and onwards, Department of Health, London.

DoH (1992a), *The Health of the Nation: a strategy for health in England,* Cmnd 1523, HMSO, London.

DoH (1992b), EL(92)47, Priorities and planning guidance 1993/4, NHSME, Department of Health, London.

DoH (1992c) *First Steps for the NHS,* NHSME, Department of Health, London.

DoH (1992d) Health at Work, NHSME, Department of Health, London.

DoH (1992e), EL(92)89, The information management and technology strategy for the NHS in England: getting better with information, NHSME, Department of Health, London.

DoH (1992f) *Developing Information Systems for Purchasers,* Information Management Group, Department of Health, London.

DoH (1992g), *Handbook for IM&T Specialists,* Information Management Group, NHSME, Department of Health, London

Earl, M.J. (1989), *Management Strategies for Information Technology,* Prentice Hall International, Hemel Hempstead, England.

Feeny, D.F., Edwards, B.R., Earl, M.J. (1987) 'Complex organisations and the information systems function. A research study', Oxford Institute of Information Management, Discussion Paper (RDP 86/10), Templeton College, Oxford.

Frost, B. and Sillince, J. (1992) 'Management information for primary care prescribing', *Journal of Management in Medicine,* 6 (4), 21-33.

Hamley, J.G., Brown, S.V., Crooks, J. (1981), 'Duplicate prescriptions: an aid to research and review', *Journal of the Royal College of General Practitioners,* 37, 531-532.

Hepburn, A. (1992) 'Indicative prescribing scheme - 1st birthday: celebration or wake?', *Practice Management,* Summer, 2,3, 36-38.

HMSO (1990), *The Exmouth Care Card Evaluation Report,* HMSO, London.

McFarlan, F.W., McKenny, J.L. (1983), *Corporate Information Systems Management: the Issues Facing Senior Executives,* Dow Jones Irwin.

Malone-Lee, M. (1992). Reported in: *NHSME News,* 58, 2-3.

Manser, P. (1992), 'Capturing quality data: behind bars', *British Journal of Health Care Computing,* September, 30-31.

Mooney, G., Healey, A., (1991), 'Strategy full of good intentions', Smith, R. (ed), *The Health of the Nation: the BMJ view,* British Medical Journal, London, 210-213.

Pringle, M., (1992), 'From theory to practice in general practice audit', *Quality in Health Care*, 1, Supplement, S12-S14.

Sandiford, P., Annett, H., Cibulski, R. (1992), 'What can information systems do for primary health care? An international perspective', *Social Science and Medicine*, 34, 1077-1087.]

Sillince, J.A.A., Frost, C.E.B. (1992), 'Information systems without a strategy: computerising British primary health care management', Sheffield University Management School, Discussion Paper (92.39), Management School, Sheffield University.

Smith, R. (1991) 'First steps towards a strategy for health', Smith, R. (ed), *The Health of the Nation: the BMJ view*, British Medical Journal, London, 1-9.

Tricker, R.I. (1982), *Effective Information Management*, Beaumont Executive Press.

Wijay, L. (1992) 'Capturing quality data: winning the paper chase', *British Journal of Health Care Computing*, September, 32.

APPENDIX 1

The IS developments promised as a result of *Promoting Better Health* and *Working for Patients* (DoH 1987 1989) provide further examples of IS developments mainly falling into the Sweetmeats category:

Action in hand following *Promoting Better Health* included:

- the FHSA Computer Evaluation Project was established to identify information required to support the business function and planning role of FHSAs in the 1990s
- FHSAs were to provide and assist GPs in providing better information for their consumers (i.e. patients)
- FHSAs were to monitor referral rates and patterns of GPs (utilising GPs' Annual Reports).

Action in hand following *Working for Patients* included:

- the role of community pharmacy IS is to be investigated.
- software supporting GP fundholders' monthly and annual reports to FHSAs is to be specified.
- shared population registers (based on FHSA patient registers) using the NHS number as the 'common patient identifier' are to be set up.
- a Data Communications Network (DCN) linking FHSA Registers with the NHS Central Register is to be established.

Following publication of Working for Patients, Framework for Information Systems: The Next Steps and Working for Patients, Framework for Information Systems: Overview (DoH 1990b, 1990c), immediate action was promised on:

- establishing RHA/FHSA information requirements regarding the Indicative Prescribing Scheme
- investigating community pharmacy requirements
- determining the details of aggregate returns from GP fundholders (to monitor expenditure against activity)
- updating the standard GP referral slip
- re-examining the proposal for encounter letters for GP fundholders.

In addition the Committee for Regulating Information Requirements will specify minimum data set changes via Data Set Change Notices. This will include the establishment of a system for GPs' and consultants' codes.

5 GP Fundholding — A Financial Management Perspective

JOHN ROBINSON, DAVID WAINWRIGHT,
JOHN NEWTON & MICHELLE FRASER
Newcastle Business School, University of Northumbria at Newcastle

INTRODUCTION

One of the main thrusts of recent government health care policy is that of devolved management of resources. This has come about as result of government trying to contain escalating costs and yet at the same time endeavouring to maintain and improve healthcare provision.

Fundholding was introduced in 1991 and provided GPs with the opportunity to manage funds which previously they had committed but for which they were not directly responsible. These funds were in respect of hospital services and prescribing. Practice management funds were already under their control.

Another substantial change affecting fundholding GPs was that of the introduction of a limited market economy — they would be able to contract directly with healthcare providers.

GPs in favour of the changes saw an opportunity to impact directly on access to, and the quality of, secondary care and in addition budget savings would benefit their practice. Patients would benefit directly from both improved hospital and practice services.

Those opponents of the scheme believed that a commercial orientation to heathcare provision would result in GPs making decisions in which financial factors carried a considerable weighting. Traditional healthcare ethics would in some way be compromised. Treatments would become commercial transactions.

An issue of concern to many people was that the emphasis on fund management would lead to the avoidance of costly patients and the employment of less costly but less effective treatments. In addition opponents of the scheme envisaged the emergence of a two tier system — if there were winners then there would be losers.

Cynics envisaged fundholders receiving larger budget allocations in order to ensure success and thereby confirm the government's approach to fund management.

Managerial Issues in the Reformed NHS. Edited by M.Malek, P.Vacani, J.Rasquinha & P.Davey
© 1993 John Wiley & Sons Ltd

As yet there is little empirical evidence to support these views. The findings of this research project support the improvement in healthcare provision but anecdotal evidence suggests that some over funding may have occurred and indeed Virginia Bottomly appears to confirm this view when stating that GPs are morally bound to repay surpluses where they are as a result of inaccuracies in setting funding levels. She went on to say that deficits would be funded.

This paper is the result of a study aimed to describe the experiences of 10 fundholding practices in the Northern region during the first year of the scheme (1991-2). This paper examines the financial management of practice funds, specifically in relation to—

- Fund allocation
- Effective management of funds
- Hospital and drug costs used in treatment decisions
- Changing referral patterns as a consequence of financial considerations

SAMPLE SIZE

A sample of nine practices was randomly selected from a list of fundholders stratified by the nine family health service authority areas in the Northern region. In one case two practices had joined the scheme as joint budget holders (a consortium), making a total of 10 in the sample.

DATA COLLECTION

Three forms of data collection were used. They were first piloted in another fundholding practice.

Firstly, two semi-structured interviews were held at each practice with the lead clinician involved in fundholding and the practice manager between February and July 1992. Each audio taped session lasted between one to one and a half hours. The first interview asked about becoming a fundholder; budget and contractual arrangements for 1991—2; impact on clinical practice; and impact on practice organisation and management. The second interview asked about the situation at the year end 1991—2; the budget for 1992—3; contracts for 1992—3, management and organisational changes; patient services; information handling; and fundholding in the next three to four years.

Secondly questionnaires were developed for self completion by other clinicians and non-medical staff in the practice. These aimed to elicit individual views about fundholding and details of the impact that it had on their roles. Clinicians were asked about the perceived costs and benefits of fundholding; involvement in fundholding; the impact of fundholding on work and relationships with consultants and others; use of information technology; and feedback from patients. Non-medical staff were asked about their involvement in the decision to apply for fundholding status; perceived costs and benefits; and the impact of fundholding on work, uses of computers, and patients. The questionnaires were designed so that responses would be given in one of three ways: a yes/no answer; a comment; or a choice from either three or five possible responses.

Thirdly a schedule was distributed to practice managers asking for information about the practice. This information was used to construct a profile of each practice.

DATA ANALYSIS

The audio taped interviews were transcribed with a word processing package. Alongside this a freeform database enabled the creation of a set of topic headings under which summarised answers from each transcript could be listed. Within each topic heading the listed answers were then further coded to determine groupings of like answers. This computer assisted process of summarising and coding made a large amount of semi-structured material amenable to qualitative analysis

Information from the structured questionnaire was entered onto computer spreadsheets. Simple statistical analysis of the spreadsheets resulted in totals and percentages of responses to each questions for each practice. Comments and responses to the practice profile questionnaire were analysed with a more structured database program.

Data collection covered many faces of fundholding; not all data was considered of relevance to financial management and so for the purposes of this paper some has been ignored. The complete data set forms the base for papers already published and in progress.

RESULTS

Allocation and agreement of budgets for 1991-2

For hospital services the data set on which the 1991—2 budgets were calculated was based on practice statistics for the 3 months immediately prior to fundholding and an estimate of the following three months activities. This data set was then extrapolated to provide annual statistics. In all practices but one there was insufficient data; also data was unreliable resulting in an inaccurate data set. Extrapolation of this data set meant that annualisation was also inaccurate. It was not possible to ascertain the degree of inaccuracy and as a consequence the degree to which funds had been over or under allocated for the year. The data set policy (3 months prior and 3 months post going live) was that of the Northern region.

For prescribing costs and practice management accurate data from the Prescription Pricing Authority PACT database was available resulting in a reliable allocation of funds.

In all cases the lead fundholding clinician and the practice manager were involved in the budget allocation process. 51% of the remainder of the clinicians were involved to a small degree. For 1992—3 the percentage of those with a low level of involvement fell to 40%.

Effective management of funds

In all cases the lead fundholding clinician and the practice manager were involved in the day to day management of funds, 54% of the other clinicians were involved to a small degree.

In all cases monthly budget reviews of hospital services, prescribing and practice administration took place. Practice administration reviews had taken place for many years in all practices and were considered reliable. Prescribing reviews were considered reliable but for hospital services they were rendered almost worthless because of a number of reasons:

- Data from providers was inaccurate and received late; there were many queries.
- Software was unable to link activities with costs.
- Software was unable to provide detailed information on individual provider contracts nor deal with outstanding cases.
- Provider unit software and practice software was incompatible.

In three instances a misunderstanding as to the nature of a provider contract resulted in a substantial miss management of funds. The contract was believed to be Block when in fact it was Cost and Volume. There was evidence that in several cases, where treatments had not been undertaken by providers during the year despite the fact that block fees were paid in full, payments for treatments would have to be duplicated in the next financial year. One practice undertook reviews by a detailed comparison of activity by activity, without any reference to costs.

The analysis of annual budget saving/overspends, (Table 1) shows that 67% of practices were able to achieve surpluses. These totalled £413,508, being 2.9% of the total annual budget allocation; of these one, for £194,392, skews the results. Adjusting for this results in annual surpluses of 1.7%. Three practices incurred deficits of between £16,500 and £50,526, in total £107,016. Overall surpluses of 2.2% were achieved.

Table 1. Budgetary Outcomes for 1991/92

Practice No	List Size	Total Budget £	Budget per Patient £	Saving (Overspend) £	Outcome as % of Total Budget
1	10,500	1,744,347	169.98	(40,000)	-2.25
2	9,712	1,463,598	150.70	46,000	3.14
3 * consortia					
4 * consortia	16,835	2,023,100	120.17	21,116	1.04
5	10,500	1,270,445	120.99	(16,500)	-1.30
6	14,000	1,673,600	119.54	63,000	3.76
7	12,500	1,555,475	124.44	61,000	3.92
8	9,900	1,399,999	141.41	47,000	3.36
9	10,800	1,511,511	139.95	194,392	12.86
10	13,900	1,637,448	117.80	(50,516)	-3.09

Hospital and drug costs used in treatment decisions

All clinicians stated that treatment costs did not form any part of the decision when referring patients. However fundholding had brought to their attention the cost of treatments.

All practices carefully monitored prescribing costs and were already moving towards greater use of generic drugs. This was not as a consequence of fundholding.

Changing referral patterns as a consequence of financial considerations

There was no evidence to suggest that referrals had changed as a consequence of financial considerations. In fact referral patterns had not changed. The reasons for this appear to be —

•   practices were loyal to their local hospitals, and;
•   Region had advised a continuation of existing relationships.

One practice was so dissatisfied with local provision that a substantial change in referrals occurred.

DISCUSSION

Perceptions of costs and benefits indicate that fundholding (see Table 2), has resulted in improvements to health care provision. The study shows that financial management was weak in all practices and therefore cannot be considered to be a major contributing factor. Having said this GPs are aware of the influence that fundholding has empowered them with and have used this directly to change relationships between consultants and provider units. The nature of contracts for 1992—3 have changed and there is little doubt that fund management will result in a realignment of referrals patterns with a subsequent redistribution of funds between provider units.

Evidence (GP statements) refutes the suggestion that financial considerations have compromised GP ethics . An in-depth study of referral patterns would be required to substantiate this statement.

GP fundholders have obtained improvements in health care provision and yet many media reports suggest deteriorating provision. This may support an emergence of a two tier system.

Because of the unreliability of data sets used in the initial allocation of funds the project team was unable to confirm that surpluses achieved during 1991—2 were as a result of good management.

Table 2. Perceptions of costs and benefits of fundholding

Benefits	No of times mentioned
General Practitioners	
Improved management and computer systems	10
Improved quality of hospital care	8
Enhanced dialogue with consultants and managers	7
Freedom of referral	5
Improved access to hospital services	5
More scrutiny of clinical practice	4
Clarification of practice goals	2
Sharing ideas with other fundholders	2
Non Medical Staff	
Swifter referrals	11
More health promotion	10
More services available to patients	8
Greater choice of hospitals	7
Better care for patients	6
More auditing of clinical work	2
Costs	
General Practitioners	
Increased time and effort in administration	14
Increased stress	3
Worsening of relations with other practitioners	2
Frustration with computer system	2
Disenchantment with ancillary staff	2
Potential for conflict with other partners	1
Non Medical Staff	
Extra work	19
Stress, disharmony and dissension	3
Loss of GP surgery time	2
Anxiety about the future	2
Less personal attention to patients	2
Widening division between doctors and nurses	1

GPs did regard these surpluses as resulting from efficient management and expect that their practices will receive the benefit. If Region claws back these surpluses (there is still some doubt) then it is likely that GPs will become disillusioned and the long-term survival of the scheme put in jeopardy. Region and government must give serious consideration to this. In addition Region must ensure the reliable collection of data both for ongoing budget setting and for second and third wave fundholders. Evidence suggests that budgets for 1992—3 were prepared on the same basis as for 1991—2. If this is the case then these problems will recur.

Fund management is carried out by a small management team consisting of the lead fundholding clinician and the practice manager. During this first year considerable pressure has been place on these individuals in terms of time and appropriate skills. These issues have to be addressed through better training and resources.

Unreliable information from provider units has resulted in ineffective operational reviews. Systems to overcome this problem are being developed. This must be done as a matter of urgency.

Software, whilst approved by the Health Service, has proved inadequate in many respects. Development work must be undertaken and supported by government. In addition government must establish strategies to ensure the integration of IT Systems between providers and purchasers.

There is little doubt that fundholding has been successful in the ten practices which form the base of this study. This would seem to be confirmed by the considerable numbers of second and third wave fundholding practices. If success is to be sustained then government must recognise that further support for better information systems, training and in some cases resources, is essential.

REFERENCES

Berg BL (1989), Qualitative research methods. Needham Heights, MA Allyn and Bacon.

Bevan G, Holland W, Mays N (1989), Working for which patients and at what cost? Lancet,(i) 947-9.

Brazier JE, Normand CEM (1991), An economic review of the NHS white paper. Scottish Journal of Political Economy, 38:96-105

Crump BJ, Cubbon MF, Hawkes R, Marchment MD (1991), Fundholding in general practice and financial risk. BMJ, 302:1582-4.

Dinwall R, Hughes D (1991), Joe Stalin and the NHS revolution. Health Service Journal , 101:23-4.

Drummond M, Hawkes R, Marchment M (1990), General practice fundholding. BMJ, 301: 1288-9.

Forbes JT (1989), Practice budgets - lifting the veil of ignorance. J R Coll Gren Pract, 39:355-86.

Glennerster H, Matsaganis M, Owens P (1992), A foothold for fundholding. London: King's Fund Institute, Research report No 12.

Glynn JJ, Murphy MP, Perkins DA (1992), GP practice budgets: an evaluation of the financial risks and rewards. Financial Accountability and Management, 8:149-61

Melzer D (1992), Supermarket fantasies. Health Service Journal, 102:17.

Mullem PM (1990), Which internal market? The NHS white paper and internal markets. Financial Accountability and Management, 6:33-50.

Newton J, Fraser M, Robinson JJ, Wainwright D (1993), Fundholding in Northern Region: the first year. BMJ, 306:375-378.

Roland M (1991), Fundholding and cash limits in primary fundholding. BMJ, 303:171-2.

Weiner J, Ferris P (1990), GP budget holding in the UK: lessons from America. London: King's Fund Institute, Research report No.7.

6 Pricing Acute Health Care in the NHS Internal Market — An Exploratory Study

SHEILA ELLWOOD

Aston Business School

INTRODUCTION

In 1989 the UK Government announced wide-ranging reform of the NHS (DoH, 1989a) which resulted in the introduction of an internal market in healthcare on 1 April, 1991. The separation of the purchasers and providers of healthcare within the NHS and the introduction of contractual arrangements, has made it imperative that healthcare products are clearly defined, costed and priced. This paper firstly considers the role of pricing in the NHS internal market, and then uses information obtained in a research study, undertaken in the year prior to the introduction of the internal market and its first year of limited operation, to assess how cost information could be improved to enhance the efficiency of the internal market.

THE NHS INTERNAL MARKET

In the internal market, district health authorities (DHAs) contract with hospitals to provide specified services in return for agreed funding. To facilitate competition between hospitals, the government introduced a number of self-governing trusts (DoH, 1989b), most hospitals now hold trust status. Although still part of the NHS, these hospitals are free from control by DHAs and operate as self standing business units. Trust hospitals and directly managed hospitals earn their revenue according to the services they supply rather than the previous global allocation. Contract funding brings about an effective separation of health authority functions: the responsibility for ensuring that the health needs of the population are met (i.e. the commissioning role) and, the management of supply. Whilst existing district health authorities are the main purchaser, at least in the short run, large GP practices have the opportunity to become budget holders to purchase selected hospital services (DoH,1989d). Similarly to DHA purchasers, the GP fund holder (GPFH) contracts with providers of healthcare for their services on behalf of the practice's patients. In the future private patients and insurance plans may figure increasingly as purchasers of services.

The Government described three forms of contract, DoH (1989c): block contracts; cost and volume contracts; and cost per case contracts. Block contracts relate to funding a level of capacity; cost and volume contracts specify a base-line level of activity, beyond that level purchasers can link payment with agreed activity; cost per case contracts cover the cost of treatment for specific patients. In addition, hospitals will sometimes undertake extra-contractual referrals (ECRs). These may arise for example when a GP refers a patient to a hospital where the DHA within which the patient resides has not negotiated a contract or perhaps the patient is admitted as an emergency e.g from a motor accident to a hospital where the DHA has no contract.

Hospitals need to keep their costs, including capital and other overheads, within the income they earn from contracts, and will accordingly need to aim for realistic pricing policies...The development of the contract system will require improved management information both for pricing and for control (including monitoring performance as well as financial control). DoH (1989c) paragraph 2.15.

MARKETS, PRICING AND ECONOMIC EFFICIENCY

Markets and economic efficiency

The concept of an internal market for healthcare in the UK had been propounded some years earlier by an American economist who saw its principle advantage as that:

> "managers would then be able to use resources most efficiently. They could buy services from producers who offered good value." Enthoven (1985: 40)

The internal market has been called a quasi-market (Le Grand 1991) as it differs from conventional markets on both the demand and the supply sides. On the supply side there is competition between service suppliers. However, these organizations are not necessarily out to maximize their profits. On the demand side, the immediate consumer is not the one who exercises the choices concerning purchasing decisions, these choices are delegated to a third party (DHA/GP) who act as a guardian of the patient's interests. Quasi-market contracts are designed to improve the efficiency of service delivery. The market will not establish allocative efficiency in the sense of determining the total amount to be spent on healthcare, but the market could aid purchasers (DHAs and GPFH) to distribute the limited NHS resources in a manner which maximizes patient welfare within the budget constraint.

The natural outcome of perfect markets is efficient behaviour - consumer satisfaction maximised at least cost to society. A market is basically an adjustment mechanism for supply and demand which enables the exchange of goods and services between consumers and producers. Markets adjust using price signals. At the given market price, producers offer their products for sale and consumers spend their disposable income according to their desires. In a perfect market no producers or consumers are left unsatisfied by the resultant exchange and distribution; at the given market price producers are able to sell all that they want (so maximising their profits) and consumers are able to purchase all they wish (so maximising their utility). If market forces lead to the achievement of a societal objective of utility maximization, it would be desirable to leave markets unfettered by government intervention.

However, for many goods free markets cannot achieve utility maximization as the conditions for a perfect market do not exist: certainty; no externalities; perfect knowledge on the part of the consumer; consumers to act free of self-interested advice from suppliers; and several small suppliers to promote genuine competition. All of these conditions are lacking in relation to healthcare (Le Grand and Robinson 1984, Mc Guire et al 1988, Mooney 1992, Donaldson and Gerard 1983). Therefore healthcare cannot be allocated efficiently under a free market system, but that is not to say that competition, managed appropriately, cannot be an important stimulus to improved efficiency.

There are undoubtedly inefficiencies within the NHS, not surprisingly in an organisation spending over £27bn per annum. Most efficiency gains are likely to arise from improvements in technical efficiency: reductions in X-inefficiency (divergence between actual and minimum cost): lower costs from economies of scale and reductions in input prices. Inefficiencies have been highlighted in a number of studies: National Audit Office 1987, Yates 1987, Audit Commission 1990 and 1991. Wagstaff concluded in 1989 that hospitals have a U-shaped cost function with minimum costs reached at 430 beds or more, suggesting scope for lower costs from economies of scale (Wagstaff, 1989). Further efficiency gains may be achieved by reductions in input prices (Bartlett and Le Grand, 1992). However, the objective of increasing the efficiency of the NHS will only be realised if the market is fed appropriate price signals.

Pricing

In purely competitive markets, the manager has no power over price, being compelled to accept the prevailing one, since price is determined by the interaction of all buyers and sellers. However, the NHS internal market is inevitably after many years of central planning, characterized by local monopolies.

> "Although there is probably a high degree of competition for services such as elective surgery, where many patients are prepared to travel, and for other services in densely populated urban areas, there will be considerable monopoly or oligopoly power in some services outside conurbations and for regional and supra regional services."
> Department of Health 1989e, EL (89) MB/171, para 7(i).

Without regulation, pricing would be subject to abuse by monopoly suppliers at least in the short run. Even in the long run, financial and other barriers to entry deter new hospitals from setting up in competition with established ones and therefore contestable markets may be difficult to ensure. Consequently, pricing methods must be designed which prevent the abuse of monopoly power if the internal market is to encourage economic efficiency. Two possible pricing approaches are a central price schedule and pricing according to the NHS provider's full cost (either through retrospective reimbursement or prospective pricing).

A central price schedule could be imposed by central government. Contracts would then be negotiated for the volume of cases to be treated in a given period and for the quality or amenity characteristics of care. In the USA, fixed-rate reimbursement has been a feature of the Medicare system since 1983. A number of studies in the USA have shown reductions in the length of hospital stays following the introduction of the Medicare fixed rate schedule (Rosko and Broyles 1987, Guterman and Dobson 1986, Kahn et al 1990). However, although a fixed-rate payment schedule may be successful in reducing the cost per patient, it cannot be used to enhance competition or to reduce the importance of non-price competition. Evidence from the USA proves that non price competition in healthcare leads, not to reduced cost and enhanced efficiency, but to excess capacity, duplication of services, increased levels of amenity and higher costs (Robinson and Luft, 1985). Schedule rates would generate cost savings only for those hospitals where the fixed rate is less than current costs. One possible response would be for hospitals to change the classification of patients into more lucrative treatment categories, a practice known as 'DRG creep' in the USA where it is prevalent (Carter and Ginsberg, 1985). A central price schedule could not be used to encourage economic efficiency in the NHS internal market as prices would not guide purchasers (DHAs and GPFH) to their most productive use and reward cost effective services. One of the ways in which monopoly rents are captured by monopolists, especially non-profit making ones, is via cost increases. If these become embodied in schedule rates, then 'average' X-inefficiency is not penalised, thus nullifying one of the main potential benefits of enhanced competition.

An alternative approach is to base contract prices on individual provider cost, either retrospective or prospective. Under a system of retrospective reimbursement at full cost, a hospital subsequently receives payment in full from purchasers for all reasonable expenditure incurred. Experience in the USA has shown that retrospective reimbursement encourages long lengths of hospital stay, excessive diagnostic testing etc. (Rosko and Broyles 1987, Guterman and Dobson 1986, Kahn et al 1990). Such a system promotes inefficiency and cost escalation, it would be extremely difficult for purchasers to keep within cash-limited allocations. A system which bases prices on prospective provider cost, on the other hand would provide greater control whilst still enabling purchasers to be guided by price. The NHSME's decision therefore to instruct NHS providers to set prices equal to prospective cost plus a rate of return on capital (NHSME, 1990) seems a rational approach. Purchasers will be guided by price to the most 'efficient' provider and providers will be encouraged to improve efficiency (as long as markets are contestable, Baumol et al 1982). However, in order to reduce the likelihood that in monopoly situations, cost-plus pricing will encourage cost-enhancing inefficiency, openness in costing and pricing is required. Culyer and

Posnett (1990) see such openness as a method of providing yardsticks to enable purchasers to assess contracts more fully. Prices should be reliable indicators of efficiency so as to feed the right signals to the market to achieve economic efficiency. In other words, prices must adequately reflect the cost of resources consumed in providing healthcare products.

COST-BASED PRICING — EXISTING INFORMATION AND THE MARKET'S NEEDS

Cost information

The NHS had operated cost and budgetary systems since its earliest days, but designed primarily to ensure probity, control total expenditure and provide data to the Department of Health rather than to facilitate pricing or to assess product cost recovery (Ellwood, 1990). Financial reporting and management accounting had developed considerably in the previous twenty years. In the early decades of the NHS, cost analysis was limited to an analysis of actual costs by subjective expenditure categories (medical supplies and equipment; drugs; uniforms etc.).

In 1974, in line with the change in organizational structures, the analysis of costs shifted to a functional basis i.e. specialized professional services e.g. nursing, pharmacy etc. and functional budgets were introduced to help monitor compliance with budget limits by heads of functions. In recent years, the development of more sophisticated costing and budgeting has been supplementary to this basic control (Perrin, 1988).

Interest in extending cost analysis down to the level of the clinician (the ultimate decision-maker on the use of NHS resources) was promulgated in the 1970s (Hillman and Nix, 1982). However it was not until 1984, that the introduction of specialty costing as a minimum for all health authorities was recommended, DHSS (1984). Specialty costing returns provided by many DHAs were not compiled as part of a continuous specialty costing system: apportionments were frequently based on sample data and were carried out only annually. The specialty costs produced only applied to "direct patient care services" rather than total hospital costs. Specialty cost returns were the lowest level of cost information which health authorities were required to provide in 1989. The costs were only required to be produced for each DHA rather than each hospital and were not included in performance indicators published by the Department of Health. However, there were a number of national and local initiatives providing more detailed information at individual hospitals, the most notable of which was the Resource Management (RM) Initiative.

The cost information available in the NHS had developed rapidly in the years prior to the Reforms, but there was very little information available at the level needed for pricing contracts, especially cost and volume and cost per case contracts.

COST ACCOUNTING APPROACHES FOR PRICING IN THE NHS INTERNAL MARKET

The DoH's approach on the pricing of contracts was set out by the NHS Management Executive in October, 1990. The fundamental principles are: contracts should generally be priced at cost, all costs including depreciation at current cost and 6% interest on capital assets should be included; and there should be no planned cross-subsidisation. Hospitals have considerable freedom to determine the product level at which costs should be attributed and to determine appropriate means of cost allocation and apportionment.

An essential feature of any market is a clear and unambiguous definition of the product to be traded. An important determinant of overall hospital costs, (in addition to the volume of services) is the range of services to be offered. The NHS Management Executive recommended specialty-based, block contracts for the majority of providers in 1991/92 (largely because of difficulties in obtaining more detailed pricing and monitoring). However, 113 procedures, investigations and out-patient visits were prescribed for pricing GPFH contracts. In the longer term, if the internal market is to achieve efficiencies through the contracting environment, contracts will have to be related to patient volume and case-mix.

Thus a classification of case-mix which condenses the infinite variety of hospital patients into appropriate groups is required. From the point of view of cost accounting, the crucial test of an appropriate product definition is the ability to define the likely resource consumption of the patient. Individual clinical specialties cover a wide range of hospital treatments from those undertaken as a day-case with little resource input to those requiring many weeks of hospital stay and high usage of resources. Specialty cases whilst initially having the practical advantage of being relatively easy to cost and therefore price would not enable resource consumption to be clearly defined and would be an unsatisfactory level at which to contract. Contracting on a specialty in-patient day as opposed to specialty case would build in a crude adjustment for case-mix within specialty, the more complex cases generally requiring longer lengths of stay. However, the difficulty of ensuring that lengths of stay are justified would require strong utilisation review and patient management.

Patient classifications based on diagnosis can be expected to synthesise the patient's symptoms and determine expected treatment. Standardised classifications of diagnoses have been available for many years through the World Health Organisation ICD schemes. Future product lines could be based on diagnosis related groups (DRGs) developed in the USA for the Medicare prospective payment system. In Britain, the evaluation of DRGs has been in progress since 1982, Sanderson et al (1989). The National Case Mix Office is currently redefining DRGs to form Healthcare Resource Groups (HRGs) for British clinical practice.

Patient grouping for contracts could, alternatively, be based on patient treatment patterns rather than diagnosis, such groupings would be particularly strong from the point of view of internal management control, but would have the disadvantage of not being readily available from existing patient coding and requiring considerable development work. Patient treatment plans would fit the cost accounting "industrial" model most closely. Variances could be measured according to the differences from planned treatment. However, whilst treatment profiles have considerable merit from the point of view of cost accounting, the numerous plans will be difficult to form into viable packaging arrangements (product lines).

Product definition and quality of services are inter-linked. Products can be differentiated on grounds of service quality; and the level of product definition also has repercussions in terms of the need for patient management and utilisation review. Ideally DHAs as the purchasers of healthcare should be concerned with health outcomes (final outputs). Existing outcome and performance measures concentrate on intermediate outputs. For example, the Queen Elizabeth Hospital (Birmingham) included in its 1991/92 contracts the following standards: generic quality standards which cover adherence to statutory standards; medical audit standards; human resource requirements; other general standards including patient and purchaser satisfaction surveys; and service specific quality standards, but re-admissions are the only final output measure included. Clearly it is important that purchasers develop and respond to further health outcome measures.

The Government White Paper, Department of Health 1989a, claimed that the internal market could operate before sophisticated cost systems were in place, but prices must be a reasonable reflection of resource consumption if the market is to facilitate an efficient allocation of NHS resources. Basically there are two methods of determining healthcare costs for pricing contracts: a top-down method of attributing costs or a bottom- up method which builds to the total cost. Initially, because of the lack of departmental costing systems, resource profiles for products and standard costing, most hospitals will use a top down approach. In the longer term, in order to reap full benefits from a cost accounting system (cost modelling, variance analysis, flexible budgeting etc.), a system which builds up the cost of intermediate products (nursing hours, theatre time, drugs, laboratory tests etc) and subsequently the cost of product lines could be developed. The bottom up approach would therefore be comparable with the industrial model for establishing product costs. Both approaches will require a costing framework which:

- Establishes the total costs of the hospital to be recovered through service income
- Identifies the volume of service to be provided
- Allocates and apportions overhead costs to treatment departments
- Attributes service costs to contracts (product lines)

The top-down approach can be implemented relatively quickly and cheaply and can easily be reconciled with actual costs. On the other hand, it will provide an imprecise measure of resource use which is likely to lack credibility and acceptability to clinicians and other healthcare professions. The extent of the imprecision will depend to a largely on the methods adopted for absorbing overheads and attributing direct service department costs to contracts. The bottom up approach would provide the most precise measure of cost and be more likely to gain acceptance with clinicians. It would also assist medical audit, the quality review process and the introduction of flexible budgeting. However, it will be much more expensive; labour intensive to develop and take considerably longer to introduce.

THE WEST MIDLANDS SURVEY — CONTRACT PRICES AND COST METHODS 1991/92

Many restrictions were placed on the operation of the internal market when it was introduced on 1 April 1991. Contracts were to be on the whole block contracts and, for DHAs, were to reflect existing referral patterns; they were to be negotiated mainly at specialty level for DHAs although each hospital had to produce prices at clinical procedure level for GPFHs, NHS Management Executive (1990d). A database of the 1991/92 prices quoted by acute hospitals in the West Midlands Region, (the largest of the fourteen health regions in England), was compiled. In order to assess the basis of the prices, a questionnaire on the costing methods used and the market environment was distributed to the financial managers of 49 acute hospitals in the Region of which 40(80%) responded.

1991/92 Healthcare Prices in the West Midlands

The database included GPFH procedure prices and extra-contractual referral (ECR) prices throughout the West Midlands Region. Hospitals had been instructed that ECR prices should be constructed on the same basis as mainstream contracts, and therefore ECR prices should be indicative of contract prices.

The database revealed vast variations in the specialty prices as shown in Table 1.

Table 1. Speciality Prices 1991/92 — West Midlands Region

ECR Prices Speciality	Price per Consultant episode			CV*
	Average £	High £	Low £	%
General medicine	1160	1472	923	14
Paediatrics	767	1139	371	27
Dermatology	1830	3417	469	59
General surgery	1148	1477	713	16
Urology	985	1714	595	30
Orthopaedics	1493	2311	854	23
ENT	754	1203	457	27
Opthalmology	934	1483	518	27
Gynaecology	635	915	443	22
Obstetrics	761	1353	350	36

* CV = coefficient of variation. Source: Cost Methods for NHS Healthcare Contracts, Ellwood (1992)

Depending on which hospital in the Region is selected, a consultant episode can cost from £350 to £1353 in obstetrics and from £469 to £3417 in dermatology and so on. For the internal market to operate satisfactorily such price differentials must be indicative of efficiency and/ or quality. However, the choice of clinical specialty as the cost product is bound to give rise to distortions due to differences in case-mix or complexity between hospitals. Specialty costs are generally believed to be at too high a level of aggregation of clinical work to be meaningful as resource groups.

Table 2. GP Fundholder Prices for General Surgery Procedures in West Midlands Health Region

Procedure		Average £	High £	Low £	Range £	CV %
General Surgery						
Partial Thyroidectomy	35	1079	1732	709	1023	23
Total Thyroidectomy	36	1284	2602	709	1893	36
Aberrant Thyroid Gland	37	945	1920	231	1689	36
Salivary Gland	38	714	958	176	782	26
Parathyroid Gland	39	1087	1819	425	1394	25
Oesophagoscopy	40	370	1057	91	966	58
Dilation of Oesophagus	41	592	3829	175	3654	117
Operation on Oesphagus	42	1623	3079	175	2904	62
Gastractomy	43	2882	6531	958	5573	40
Vagotomy	44	1584	3504	775	2729	38
Endoscopy	45	359	1106	91	1015	67
Laparoscopy	46	370	577	188	389	28
Small Intestine lesion	47	1567	3261	869	2392	32
Part Colectomy	48	2510	3668	958	2710	26
Total Colectomy	49	2772	4968	958	4010	27
Sigmoidoscopy	50	568	1121	91	1030	56
Colonoscopy	51	448	958	136	822	52
Ext. of Bowel	52	2399	5474	527	4947	44
Prolapsed rectum	53	1780	2897	922	1975	31
Anal Fissure	54	554	1007	91	916	43
Rectum excision	55	2899	5503	958	4545	32
Pilonidal sinus	56	785	2128	459	1669	45
Dilation of anal sphincter	57	320	958	91	867	56
Haemorrhoidectomy	58	782	1276	213	1063	29
Gall bladder	59	1408	2536	638	1898	32
Bile ducts	60	2193	3794	958	2836	29
Masectomy	61	1382	2464	637	1827	33
Breast lesion	62	497	1277	231	1046	44
Inguinal hernia	63	671	1795	303	1492	43
Femoral hernia	64	778	1719	351	1368	40
Incisional hernia	65	1295	2433	175	2258	37
Varicose veins	66	544	1278	287	991	38
Ingrowing toenail	67	236	656	91	565	44
Skin biopsy	68	363	1165	91	1074	64
Lymph node excision	69	518	958	213	745	35

Source: Cost Methods for NHS Healthcare Contracts, Ellwood (1992)

The USA and many European and Scandinavian countries prefer to use diagnostic related groups (DRGs), as indeed has the NHS in its resource management approach, to classify patients into types that are similar both clinically and in the resources they use. It was therefore expected that less variation would be found in procedure costs as procedures are broadly in line with DRGs. However, the variation in prices of many procedures between hospitals as measured by the coefficient of variation is greater than the variation between specialty prices per episode, the analysis of general surgery procedures is shown in Table 2.

The prices quoted by NHS hospitals in the West Midlands are generally below those for fixed price surgery in private hospitals. For example, BUPA quotes a price of £1,135 for a tonsillectomy compared with a range of £143 to £958 in NHS acute hospitals in the West Midlands. The fundamental question is whether the prices quoted by NHS providers are adequate for the market mechanism to operate effectively. Does the 1991/92 price for treatment of an ingrown toe-nail at one West Midlands hospital of £91 compared with £656 at another provide the right signals to the market?

Whilst price variations are an important facet of a market system, the market will only improve resource allocation if prices fairly reflect costs, such price variations in procedures could be due to the crude nature of the costing approaches rather than true variations in treatment patterns and the cost of resource inputs. In order to assess the reliability of the prices, the questionnaire sent to acute hospitals in the West Midlands covered both the nature of the market environment (the form of contracts and the number of purchasers) and the approach to costing contracts/ ECRs and GPFH procedures.

The Market in the West Midlands

The questionnaire results showed the nature of the market to be very diverse. Of the 40 hospitals completing the questionnaire the contracting environment varied from one hospital with contracts with only 2 health authorities (Princess Royal in Shropshire) to one holding contracts with 23 health authorities (Queen Elizabeth, Birmingham). The Birmingham hospitals faced considerably more competition than the other hospitals, 9 of the 10 hospitals which contracted with more than 15 DHAs were within the city. Similarly, the number of contracts with GPFHs varied from nil at one West Midlands hospital to 16 at Birmingham Women's Hospital. The average provider hospital contracted with 10 health authorities and 2 GPFHs. An on-going research study by the National Association of Health Authorities and Trusts (NAHAT) monitoring the degree of competition in general surgery faced by hospitals in the West Midlands Region suggests that only a quarter of them operate in markets where the degree of competition is such that elements of monopoly or oligopoly power may exist, Robinson (1991).

The form of the contracts held also showed extreme diversity. The average provider hospital had the following pattern of contract income (see Table 3):

Table 3. Contract Income

	% of Contract Income
Block	28
Block with indicative volume	61
Cost and volume	8
Cost per case	3

However, 8 hospitals earned 100% of their contract income through block contracts whilst at the other extreme, one hospital earned 95% of its contract income through cost and volume contracts and 5% cost per case and another hospital 100% through cost and volume contracts.

Block contracts are specified in terms of facilities to be provided rather than explicit workload; the DHA provides resources in regular instalments, irrespective of the volume of patients treated, and for which no explicit usage is prescribed. Such contracts provide little incentive to improve efficiency. Cost and volume contracts place an explicit requirement on the provider in terms of patients treated. Often a fixed price is paid up to a volume threshold above which a price per case is set up to a volume ceiling. Cost per case contracts are obviously the most risky, the provider would have no assurity of income, whilst the purchaser would risk losing control of expenditure if large commitments on a per case basis were incurred.

In order to investigate the financial vulnerability of hospitals in the first year of the market, the hospitals were asked to categorize their income into three elements: fixed (block contracts and the floor level of cost and volume contracts); variable (cost per case contracts - ECRs, private patients) and non patient care (special funds for training etc.). In 1991/92, only 2 hospitals had more than 5% of their income classified as variable. However, given the fixed nature of most hospital costs even small percentage falls in funding can have dramatic effects, 15 hospitals classified between 2 and 4% of their income as variable. This cost structure explains the apparent zeal with which hospitals endeavour to retain or capture additional income from GPFH.

Thus the internal market poses much more of a threat/ opportunity to some hospitals than others and consequently the importance of realistic pricing and costing methods is much greater to the more market orientated hospitals.

THE COST METHODS BEHIND THE PRICES

In pricing contracts for health authorities, all 40 hospitals used a specialty cost approach although GPFH contracts and regional specialty contracts were priced at a more detailed level. Most hospitals (24 or 62%) used the annual specialty cost return as the start point, a further 4 used actual financial ledger costs and 11 used budget information.

The average cost structure of the 40 hospitals surveyed is: 61% direct patient treatment; 20% general services; 5% District HQ and Regional Health Authority services; and 14% capital charges. However, considerable variation was apparent: one hospital classified only 43% of its costs as direct patient treatment whilst another classified 78% as direct patient treatment; capital charges varied from as little as 4% to over 20% of total costs!

Establishing realistic capital charges proved particularly difficult. Indeed massive discrepancies in the estimates of capital charges across the country forced the Department of Health to effectively "write off the first year of the system as a purely paper exercise" (Health Service Journal, 5 December, 1991). Estimated figures for 1991/92 by one district in the West Midlands were almost £2m or 33% above the final charges for 1991/92. The NHS had enormous teething problems in moving from a system where the principles of capital accounting were entirely absent to one in which all assets over £1,000 were subject to a depreciation and interest charge, NAHAT, 1991. The Department of Health is to increase the threshold for capital items to £5,000 with effect from 1 April 1993, NHSME (1992).

For the average hospital, non direct patient care services account for 39% of total costs. Therefore a large proportion of healthcare costs can not be directly attributed to contracts even if contracts are defined only at specialty level. The vast majority of hospitals included such costs by an addition to in-patient and out-patient contracts rather than through a staged approach i.e assigning to direct treatment departments such as theatres, radiology etc for absorption into specialties. For some remote overheads this may be acceptable, but less than a third of hospitals assigned capital equipment to treatment departments, given the heavy capital equipment costs in some treatment departments (e.g. radiology) this must have distorted specialty costs.

The problem of achieving reasonable specialty costs and hence realistic prices was further exacerbated by the limited availability of cost systems for direct patient treatment services. None of the 40 hospitals had a case-mix management system and departmental costing systems were quite rare as shown in Table 4.

Table 4. Availability of Departmental Cost Systems 1990

	No. of hospitals	%
Nursing	6	15
Pharmacy	17	44
Theatres	6	15
Pathology	14	36
Radiology	9	23

Source: Cost Methods for NHS Healthcare Contracts, Ellwood (1992)

Thus in 1991/92, not only were overheads treated crudely, but also many direct patient care costs were assigned to contracts based on very limited financial information. Many hospitals however, stated that cost systems were now being introduced: a further 10 (25%) hospitals were installing nursing cost management systems; a further 6 (13%) theatre costing systems and a further 4 (10%) pharmacy costing systems. However, apart from pharmacy where 54% of hospitals had cost systems, departmental cost systems for attributing direct patient care costs to contracts were not available in the majority of hospitals.

Although, hospitals were compelled to produce prices at procedure level for GPFHs, most hospitals had limited information from which to compile such prices. All hospitals based the procedure costs on specialty in-patient day costs, these were modified by 54% of hospitals for prophesies; by 49% for theatre costs and by 15% for drug costs. Over 30% of hospitals made no adjustments to the specialty in-patient day cost when compiling procedure costs.

In determining their hospital costs and prices, 90% of hospitals had used linked spreadsheets designed in-house or by another DHA Changes in expected activity levels had often been treated crudely; some stated "general percentage uplift"; only 18% claimed to have made an analysis of fixed and variable components.

FEEDING THE MARKET THE RIGHT SIGNALS?

The cost methods used to price 1991/92 contracts in the West Midlands fall far short of the requirements necessary to facilitate an efficient market allocation of NHS resources. Specialty contracts provide an imprecise definition of services (product lines) - variations in case-mix within specialty are not addressed. On the other hand, where procedure prices were compiled they were often based on inadequate cost methods. Consequently, prices were not a reliable indicator of resources consumed. Price differences may be spurious; differences may be caused by difficulties in determining the prospective quantum of cost (particularly in relation to capital charges); inadequate activity measurement and poor methods of cost attribution. A high proportion of total costs were attributed to contracts on inadequate information. Even direct patient care costs at specialty level were of dubious credibility and the understanding of cost behaviour very limited. Furthermore, efficiency comparisons are hampered by a lack of consistency in cost allocation and apportionment methods between different hospitals. For some hospitals located in rural areas with little "competition" the effect of the internal market may be slight, for others the operation of realistic cost methods on which to price contracts may be crucial to their future viability under the internal market.

LESSONS FROM THE RESOURCE MANAGEMENT SITES AND THE USA

Resource Management Initiative

When the NHS reforms were announced, it was widely believed that the six RM pilot sites initiated in 1986 would provide the answer to hospitals' information needs and enable them to generate sufficiently reliable cost information to operate treatment tariffs, and enter into commercial contracts with DHAs, GPFH or other purchasers. Consequently, further hospitals were chosen as RM "roll out" sites to pilot systems which could be extended to all 260 major acute hospitals in the country. In 1986, the purpose of the RM initiative had been stated as:

> "to enable the National Health Service to give better service to its patients, by helping clinicians and other managers to make better informed judgements about how the resources they control can be used to maximum effect." DHSS 1986.

As the focus of RM had been in involving doctors and nurses in managing their resources, the greater part of the hospital budgets at the RM hospitals were attributed to clinical directorates. The extent varied between RM hospitals: at Guy's Hospital 67% of hospital expenditure was attributed to directorates; at Huddersfield Royal Infirmary all expenditure was attributed to directorates (Ellwood 1992).

The RM hospitals had invested heavily in computer systems including case-mix management systems. Indeed all the RM hospitals, except one which had still to incur its main programme of computer implementation, made over £1m investment in information systems between starting RM and the end of 1990. The hospitals had been experimenting with the use of diagnoses related groups (DRGs), but did not use DRGs or any other form of patient grouping as part of routine management. Care profiles consisting of the expected pattern of care for a given type of patient were also being developed at the RM hospitals. Although one of the original aims of RM expressed by the Department of Health and Social Security was to develop case-mix planning and costing, DHSS 1986, most RM hospitals had been slow to introduce costs into the RM database. Huddersfield Royal Infirmary held standard costs for the following events: ward cost per day; pathology test; radiology investigation; therapy recorded unit; drugs; theatre time (Ellwood, 1992). None of the RM hospitals had been able to provide budgets based on standard costs and expressed in terms of case-mix activity by consultant/ specialty.

No RM hospital used costs from the case-mix database for contracts with DHAs in 1991/92. The level of contracting did not require such information, and the figures held in the case-mix system were often not reconcilable to the total hospital costs because of incomplete or missing data (Ellwood,1992).

Hospital cost accounting in the USA

Whilst some pointers have been provided by the leading resource management sites in the UK, the feasibility of more sophisticated cost accounting approaches needed to meet internal market requirements were unproven. The USA is the only major developed economy in which health care provision is characterized by any significant degree of competition and therefore it was envisaged that the USA would provide a valuable insight into how health care could be costed for a competitive environment. However, there are marked differences between the purpose of cost accounting in the

USA and the UK. In the UK the role of cost accounting in the reformed NHS is to produce prices based on cost for contracting. If costs are "incorrect", contracting decisions are made on an erroneous basis and providers achieve unplanned under/ over-recovery of costs. In the USA, the role of cost accounting is to compare costs with reimbursement rates, (charges or for Medicare patients a fixed price per DRG). If costs are "incorrect" management information on product profitability is misleading.

Given the comparatively strong market approach to healthcare provision and purchasing in the USA, it would appear reasonable to expect hospitals to employ cost systems which clearly establish the cost of their healthcare "products". Some hospitals in the USA do have cost accounting systems which employ a standard costing approach integrated into an overall resource management context. However, industrial model systems are not the norm although their incidence is increasing (HFMA Massachusetts 1991, Counte and Glandon 1988), or as advanced as their literature suggests (Orloff et al 1990). Most hospitals impute patient costs from patient charges.

There are some excellent examples of cost accounting systems operating along business principles and integrated with the resource management approach. The New England Medical Centre (NEMC) in Boston has developed and maintained a sophisticated cost accounting system over the last ten years. The methodologies used at NEMC are based on business principles commonly used in industry e.g. responsibility centres, marginal costing, standard costing, variance analysis and sales forecasting. The costing model is shown in Table 5. Cost accounting focuses on the control and management of costs of intermediate products, this embodies identification of fixed and variable costs within each department; definition of intermediate products for subsequent costing; development of standard unit costs, indirect cost allocation/ apportionment; variance analysis and department cost simulation. NEMC is able to use the costings of intermediate products together with defined treatment protocols to establish budgets. The treatment protocols delineate the appropriate range in number and mix of services necessary for providing high quality care to a very specifically defined (homogeneous) type of patient. Comparison of actual and budgeted resource use can therefore enable meaningful variance analysis.

Whilst the NEMC has shown the technical feasibility of a sophisticated costing approach to costing health care, pragmatism is necessary when adopting such systems. The NEMC uses standards for all patient level details. However, therapy departments are often based on relative value units or included in indirect overhead. The "80/20" rule is often applied: each service item is ranked by budgeted $ volume; the 20% of the service items that are expected to account for 80% of the $ volume receive the majority of costing attention; the remaining 80% of service items representing 20% of the $ volume, are costed in a less time-consuming manner. Furthermore the costs held on patient records are uplifted by 20 to 25% to cover general overheads. No significant benefit is perceived to justify the development of complicated methods for attributing remote overheads to patients. The hospital sees its cost accounting system as increasingly important in ensuring the negotiation of viable contracts with Health Maintenance Organizations and Preferred Provider Organizations and also in assessing the true return on work undertaken under Medicare DRG reimbursement.

Table 5. The Costing Model — New England Medical Centre

Hospital Production Function	Raw Goods	Intermediate Products	End Products	Product Lines
	Labour, supplies capital	Nursing, lab tests x-rays	DRG ICD-9-CM Surgery Procedures	HMO/PPO Speciality Services
Type/Level management	Departmental		Clinical	Finance/planning/ marketing
Managerial objectives	Manage the cost of raw goods and services	Manage the unit cost of intermediate products	Manage the utilization of intermediate products	Market existing products to markets Market new products to existing markets Improve bottom line

CONCLUSIONS

The internal market could improve the efficiency of service delivery if purchasers are guided by price to the most 'efficient' provider and providers are encouraged to improve efficiency by competition or the threat of new entrants. Where the market is not contestable, openness in the costing and pricing of healthcare may provide a spur to improved efficiency. Guiding purchasers to achieve a more efficient allocation of the NHS resources requires prices to be a reasonable reflection of the cost of providing the various healthcare products. Healthcare contracts must reflect the long term costs of providing healthcare taking account of the quantity of provision and related to appropriate quality (outcome) measures. The market will not establish allocative efficiency in the sense of determining the total amount to be spent on the NHS although the contracting process could conceivably influence the level of spending by making explicit the quantity and forms of healthcare to be met from the public purse. However, purchasers should endeavour to maximise patient welfare by distributing the limited NHS funds in a manner which maximises patient welfare within the budget constraint.

In the initial years of the internal market, prices are not providing appropriate signals. Block contracts have predominated, consequently hospital income is not closely linked to activity and the familiar scene of NHS hospitals refusing to admit non urgent patients in the latter months of the financial year in order to keep within budget is still common (Public Finance and Accountancy 5/2/1993). Progress towards a preponderance of cost and volume contracts and cost per case contracts is required. Healthcare contract categories (product lines) are not defined adequately, specialty level contracts do not address the problem of case-mix within specialties and make comparisons difficult. Contract categories need to be established which divide each specialty into a manageable number of treatment groupings; these groupings should contain treatments which are reasonably similar in terms of resource use and which represent a high proportion of the total costs of the specialty. Furthermore, the cost methods adopted have not provided comparable, realistic prices for healthcare contracts.

Providers have been given considerable discretion in how costs are attributed to contracts, but the "full" cost (price) of healthcare products will vary according to the methods adopted. It is important to achieve consistency in the costing approaches and have adequate disclosure of prices and their cost elements (70% of purchasers in a recent survey reported difficulty in obtaining comparative cost data, NAHAT 1992). A consistent framework for classifying costs and assigning overhead costs needs to be specified. The West Midlands survey has shown that most providers assign many overheads direct to contracts (the simplest, but most inaccurate approach). Given the large element of overheads in healthcare, a more realistic and standardised approach should be adopted, perhaps along the lines of the "step-down" rules used in Medicare Cost Reporting in the USA, (Wise 1992).

Progress towards the industrial model of cost accounting has been achieved at RM hospitals in the UK, but establishing patient costing systems is a lengthy process. Some hospitals in the USA do have cost accounting systems which employ a standard costing approach integrated into an overall resource management context. However, industrial model, cost accounting systems for healthcare are expensive. To establish costs at patient level a case mix management system is required, (this alone has been conservatively estimated to add 1.4% to 3.3% to existing costs, Buxton et al 1991). An alternative way of achieving sub specialty costs for healthcare contract pricing would be to use relative weightings derived from patient costing systems at leading RM hospitals. However, this assumes constant relative efficiency between providers: it is precisely these differing levels of efficiency that prices are supposed to identify if they are to provide appropriate signals to purchasers. Each provider must assess the relative resource use between contract categories. Bases which fairly reflect the resource usage of treatment departments must be determined.

The diagram of the internal market continuum (Table 6) shows how contracts and cost information for pricing could be developed. Improved consistency, contract definition and bases of cost attribution must be achieved before cost-based pricing can provide reliable indicators of comparative performance and hence feed appropriate price signals to purchasers.

Table 6. The Internal Market Continuum

	1991		Mid 1990s
FORM OF CONTRACT	Block	⟶	Cost and volume Cost per case
PRODUCT DEFINITION	Speciality	⟶	Procedure (based on grouping of treatment plans)
COST METHODS			
Basic approach	Top-down	⟶	Bottom-up
Direct treatment	Few Cost	⟶	**Departmental Cost Systems**
Services	Systems		Intermediate product costs: * Determined by standards for all major direct patient treatment services * RVUs used for less significant services * Analysis of fixed & variable elements
Overheads	Allocated or apportioned according to available apportionment bases (often direct to contracts)	⟶ ⟶	**Influenced by direct patient treatment** Assigned to direct patient treatment department Included in intermediate product cost **Remote Overheads** Remain at hospital level Recovered by a percentage uplift to assigned costs
PERFORMANCE MONITORING	Limited to intermediate output measures	⟶	Systems fo measuring final outcomes Systematic Medical Audit Utilization Review Programme
	Departmental budgets	⟶	Budget structures based on product lines, flexed according to contracts. Variance analysis at procedure level.

Source: Cost Methods for NHS Healthcare Contracts, Ellwood (1992)

REFERENCES

Audit Commission (1990), A Short Cut to Better Services: Day Surgery in England and Wales, HMSO.

Audit Commission (1991), The Pathology Services: A Management Review, HMSO.

Bartlett, W. and Le Grand, J. (1992), The Impact of NHS Reforms on Hospital Costs, Studies in Decentralisation and Quasi-Markets, No.8, School for Advanced Urban Studies, University of Bristol

Baumol, W.J., Panzar, J.C. and Willig, R.D. (1982), Contestable Markets and the Theory of Industry Structure, Harecourt Brace Jovanovich, New York.

Buxton, M., Packwood,T., and Keen, J. (1991), Final Report of the Brunel University Evaluation of Resource Management, Brunel University.

Carter, G and Ginsburg, P. (1985), The Medicare Case Mix Index Increase: Medical Practice Changes, Ageing and DRG Creep, R-3292-HCFA, The Rand Corporation, Santa Monica.

Counte, M.A. and Glandon G.L. (1988), Managerial Innovation in the Hospital: An Analysis of the Diffusion of Hospital Cost Accounting Systems, Hospital and Health Services Administration, Fall 33.3 371-84

Culyer, A.J. and Posnett, J. (1990), Hospital Behaviour and Competition, Culyer et al (ed.), Competition in Health Care, MacMillan, Basingstoke.

Department of Health (1989a), Working for Patients, HMSO, London.

Department of Health (1989b), Self Governing Hospitals, Working for Patients, Working Paper No 1, HMSO, London.

Department of Health (1989c), Funding and Contracts for Hospital Services, Working for Patients, Working Paper No 2, HMSO, London.

Department of Health (1989d), Practice Budgets for General Medical Practitioners, Working for Patients, Working Paper No 3, HMSO, London.

Department of Health (1989e), EL (89) MB/171, Discussion Document on Pricing and Openness in Contracts for Health Services.

DHSS (1984), Steering Group on Health Service Information (Chairman: Mrs E. Korner) Sixth Report to the Secretary of State, HMSO, London.

DHSS (1986) Health Service Management - Resource Management (Management Budgeting) in Health Authorities, Health Notice, HN(86)34

Donaldson, C. and Gerard, K. (1993), Economics of Health Care Financing - The Visible Hand, MacMillan, London.

Ellwood, S. (1990), Competition in Healthcare, Management Accounting, 1990, April vol 68 no.4, 24-28.

Ellwood, S. (1992), Cost Methods for NHS Healthcare Contracts, CIMA, London.

Enthoven, A. (1985), Reflections on the Management of the National Health Service, Nuffield Provincial Hospitals Trust, London.

Ferguson, B. and Posnett, J. (1990), Pricing and Openness in Contracts for Health Care Services, Occasional Paper 11, Centre for Health Economics, University of York.

Guterman, S. and Dobson, A. (1986), Impact of the Medicare prospective payment system for hospitals, Health Care Financing Review, 7: 97-114.

HFMA Massachusetts Chapter USA (1991) Cost Accounting, Budgeting and Decision Support Practices in Massachusetts Hospitals. (Unpublished Survey).

Hillman, R.L. and Nix, G.R. (1983), DHSS Funded Research into Specialty Costing 1980-1982, DHSS, London.

Kahn, K.L., Rogers, W.H., Rubenstein, L.V., Sherwood, M.J., Reinisch, E.J. et al (1990), Measuring quality of care with explicit process criteria before and after implementation of the DRG based prospective payment system, Journal of the American Medical Association, 264: 1969- 1973.

Le Grand, J. (1991), Quasi-Markets and Social Policy, The Economic Journal, Vol 101 No 408 September 1991, 1256-1267

Le Grand, J. and Robinson, R. (1984), The Economics of Social Problems - The Market versus the State, McMillan Education Ltd, London.

McGuire, A., Henderson, J. and Mooney, G. (1988), The Economics of Health Care, Routledge and Kegan Paul Ltd, London.

Mooney, G. (1992), Economics, Medicine and Health Care, Harvester, Wheatsheaf, London.

NAHAT (1991), A Review of Capital Charges in the NHS: Cutting through the Confusion, NAHAT, Birmingham

NAHAT (1992), Monitoring the White Paper: Managed Competition, NAHAT, Birmingham

National Audit Office (1987), Use of Operating Theatres in the National Health Service, HMSO, London.

NHS Management Executive (1990), Costing and Pricing Contracts: Cost Allocation Principles.

NHS Management Executive (1992), FDL (92) 70.

Orloff et al (1990), Hospital Cost Accounting: Who's doing what and why, Management Review, Winter 1990.

Packwood, T., Buxton, M. and Keen, J. (1991), Hospitals in Transition, Open University Press.

Perrin, J. (1988), Resource Management in the NHS, Chapman and Hall, London.

Robinson, J. and Luft, H. (1985), Competition and the Cost of Hospital Care, Journal of the American Medical Association 1987 vol 257 23 3241- 5.

Robinson, R. (1991), Who's Playing Monopoly, Health Service Journal 28 March.

Rosko, M.D. and Broyles, R.W. (1987), Short term responses of hospitals to the DRG prospective pricing mechanism in New Jersey, Medical Care, 25: 88-99.

Sanderson, H.F., Storey, A., Morris, D., McNay, R.A., Robson, M.P. and Loeb, J. (1989), Evaluation of Diagnoses Related Groups in the National Health Service, Community Medicine Vol 11 4 269-278.

Wagstaff, A. (1989), Econometric studies in health economics: a survey of the British literature, Journal of Health Economics, Vol 8, 1-51.

Wise, J. (1992), Hospital Cost Accounting in the United States, CIPFA, London.

Yates, J. (1987), Why are we waiting? An Analysis of Hospital Waiting Lists, Oxford University Press.

7 The Main Influences of Doctor Prescribing Behaviour and the Role of Pharmaceutical Company Promotional Activity

ANN-MARIE CRAIG[1], MO MALEK[1] & PAUL BEARDON[2]
[1]*University of St. Andrews*
[2]*University of Dundee*

INTRODUCTION

Prescription drugs are a directed market in that the decision-maker, the doctor, is not the final consumer and so does not incur any costs. It is hoped that he or she will evaluate all alternatives and match the characteristics of a product to fulfil the respective requirements, a rational choice which is appropriate, safe, effective and economical. This choice process is a two stage development. The first stage is the identification of the various therapeutic options available, followed by the choice of appropriate therapy, perceived to be based on the operational characteristics of a product, namely the consideration of efficacy, adverse side-effects and ease of administration. It is at this stage that doctors can be emotionally swayed by brand loyalty, packaging, popularity and other aspects of pharmaceutical company promotional activity.

In this decision process doctors may look at each case and weigh up the pros and cons, undertaking an active means of problem solving, or they may develop a rule of thumb based on previous experience and similar cases thus arriving at habitual prescribing based on reasoned rules. There is also the possibility of habitual prescribing based on unreasoned rules were company promotional activities may have an influence (Denig & Haaijer-Ruskamp 1992). Advertising is meant to give the consumer information about the product which they can check, although the manufacturers can restrict the information reaching consumers. For example the incumbent can 'jam' channels through which entrants transmit their messages by loading the sampled population, the doctors, with messages of its own (Hurwitz and Caves 1988).

Managerial Issues in the Reformed NHS. Edited by M.Malek, P.Vacani, J.Rasquinha & P.Davey
© 1993 John Wiley & Sons Ltd

This paper aims to identify what the main influences of this prescribing decision are and what sources of information doctors use to arrive at their decisions. Within this context we hope to isolate the importance doctors place on company promotional activities to determine whether irrational decisions play a part or not.

The pharmaceutical industry is based on innovation hence the major companies incur huge research and development costs (R&D). The figure of $200 million is frequently mentioned on the cost of bringing a new drug into the market place, although the figure is constantly moving up. To earn an adequate return on their capital marketing tools are essential in securing brand loyalty for patented products to advertise their supposed superior quality, efficacy and safety. Once the patent has expired rigorous price competition from generic alternatives is possible but by concentrating marketing on the more expensive patented products it is possible to delay this via generating and sustaining brand loyalty. Thus the market share may be maintained or only fall at a minimum rate even in the face of cheaper competition. It would be possible that by choosing an expensive brand product over a cheaper equivalent irrational decisions are made with substantial cost implication for pharmacy budgets.

Methodology

211 questionnaires were sent to doctors in the Fife and Tayside regions of Scotland in September 1992. This questionnaire consisted of 15 questions designed to allow the doctor to identify the influences and sources of information which they believed to be most important in relation to the prescribing decision (see appendix). The questionnaire was also designed to determine general attitudes towards brand and generic drugs, knowledge of market competition, the extent of pharmaceutical company activities and the importance of such activation to dissemination of medical information.

The doctors were selected from regional telephone directories and the questionnaires were sent out 'blind' - without any knowledge of the date of registration or the sex of the respondent doctor,. Each questionnaire was anonymous and sent with a stamped addressed envelope to encourage completion and return. 145 questionnaires were returned giving a response rate of 69% and consisting of; 92 Pre-1980 registration, 50 1980 and after registration, 3 no registration date given

For the investigation of possible age-related differences in prescribing decisions and attitudes we used the date of registration of each doctor as a proxy for age. Considering the fact that generic competition only really took off in the late 1970's we therefore divided the doctors between those registered before 1980 and those registered in 1980 and afterwards.

In investigating the overall influences of doctor prescribing and the sources of information we used all of the returned questionnaires, but when considering the specific age-groups we considered only those responses that were dated.

PRESCRIBING INFLUENCES AND SOURCES OF INFORMATION

We specified thirteen possible influences over the prescribing decision and ten possible sources of information and asked each doctor to rank them according to the importance they placed on each factor. The ranking procedure specified was a simple numerical system with the following definitions.

Rank	Definition
1	of no influence/importance
2	interesting but of no direct use
3	useful but not an important influence
4	quite important
5	very important

We took the number of doctors and multiplied them by the rank they indicated to give an absolute value which was used to table each factor in descending order of importance. Table 1 indicates the factors which influence the prescribing decision, their most frequent rank and the percentage of doctors who chose them. It shows efficacy and previous personal experience as the two most important factors, with 79% and 66% respectively of all doctors ranking these factors as very important. These were followed by the quality of the product, the information read in medical journals, the price of the product, information from academic seminars and conferences, colleagues experiences of the product, and the formularies of the practice or local hospital, all of which were ranked as quite important. The quick recall of a product name was ranked useful, but not important, while company promotional activity was far down the list of influences, ranked interesting but of no direct use. At the bottom of the list came external pressures and spelling, with the majority of all doctors (40% and 50% respectively) viewing them as of no importance at all.

Table 1. Factors influencing prescribing decisions

Order	Factor	Most frequent rank	%
1	Efficacy of product	5	79
2	Previous personal experience	5	66
3	Quality of product	4	41
4	Information in medical journals	4	60
5	Price of product	4	46
6	Academic seminars, conferences	4	52
7	Colleague experiences	4	45
8	Patient preferences	4	39
9	Formularies of practice/hospital	4	32
10	Quick recall of product name	3	39
11	Promotional inf.. of companies	2	37
12	External pressure i.e.. health board	1	40
13	Spelling of product name	1	50

Table 2 indicates the specific sources of information in a similar format to Table 1. The most important sources of information identified by the doctors were the academic seminar and conference, and the independent scientific journal. In descending order of importance the various forms of information from the pharmaceutical companies came at the bottom of the list, especially the information acquired from advertisements in journals and company direct mail.

Table 2. Sources of Information

Order	Source of information	Most frequent rank	%
1	Academic seminars & conferences	4	52
2	Independent scientific journals	4	52
3	Patient feedback	4	49
4	Colleague experiences	4	44
5	Local drug information services	4	39
6	Formularies	4	32
7	Company sales representatives	3	42
8	Company seminars, conferences	3	42
9	Company advertising in journal	1	38
10	Company direct mailing	1	44

PHARMACEUTICAL COMPANY PROMOTIONAL ACTIVITY

Background Information

Questions were asked relating to the average number and length of visits a doctor receives from sales representatives, their specific attitudes towards brand and generic products, their knowledge of market conditions and company identities and what they thought company promotional activity did for them.

We discovered that 44% of all doctors found the complicated generic spelling of product names a deterrent to prescribing in an everyday clinic situation. This contrasted with the answer shown in Table 1 whereby the spelling of drug names was ranked as of no importance in the prescribing decision. Nevertheless 37% said they made a conscious effort to prescribe all drugs by their generic name irrespective of generic availability, while 36% preferred to prescribe brand-name drugs. Over two-thirds of our surveyed doctors had predetermined views with regards the type of drugs they preferred to prescribe.

To establish how much knowledge these doctors possessed of market competition we asked about their awareness of patent expiry dates and the entry of generic competition into the market (interpreting awareness as the year of patent expiry or generic entry) With reference to these fewer than 7% in both cases, knew of the dates of such occurrences. This is not as bad as it first seems as approximately 60% of them were aware of these 'sometimes'. A comprehensive knowledge of the market, specifically patent expiry and generic entry seems somewhat lacking. For those who prescribed generically irrespective of availability and those who preferred brands, this kind of knowledge is irrelevant, however for the remaining doctors (approximately 27%) there is a possibility of continued brand prescribing despite cheaper availability of generic alternative simply because it is unknown to the doctor. A situation which is likely to benefit the original high-profile patented product.

With reference to pharmaceutical company representative seen by the doctors, 46% were visited on average once a week by the company sales representatives and 31% more than once a week, while the most popular length of visit was 10 minutes with nearly 70% of all doctors indicating this length of time as the duration of the drug representative visit.   Although most doctors saw representatives frequently, only 33% thought that company sales representatives actually served their purpose of spreading relevant information on drugs.   59% believed the representatives 'sometimes' did their job properly. Most of the comments from the doctors relating to this question indicated that the success of company sales representatives in spreading relevant information was very much dependent on the individual sales representative, therefore these figures hold little weight in aggregate terms.

Looking at the relation between the promotional activities and doctors awareness, 84% of all doctors could identify certain therapeutic groups that experienced more aggressive promotional activity from the companies.   The six most frequently indicated therapeutic groups, in descending order of popularity were;

1.   Cardiovascular
2.   Anti-Ulcer
3.   Antibacterial
4.   Anti-Depressants
5.   Musculoskeletal
6.   Respiratory System

When asked if certain companies could be distinguished as promoting their products much more aggressively than others only 39% of the doctors responded. From their answers the most frequently indicated companies, in descending order were;

1.   Glaxo
2.   SmithKline Beecham
3.   Bayer
4.   Merck = Roche
5.   I.C.I. = Lilly

Company Promotional Activity

Looking specifically at pharmaceutical company promotional behaviour and influence, we chose to identify company sales representatives, company sponsored seminars and conferences, company advertising in journals and company direct mail to the doctors as the main tools used.

To determine the main value of such promotional activities as a source of information we suggested four possibilities and asked doctors to rank them as before. The results are shown in Table 3, where company promotional material and activities are indicated as primarily used for learning about new products, then new dosages, formulations and indications, reminders of existing products and finally learning about new advances in research for future reference.

Table 3. The Type of Information Provided by Company Promotional Activity

Order	Type of information	Most frequent rank	%
1	Learn of new products	4	46
2	Learn of new indications, dosages etc.	3	42
3	Reminders of existing products	3	40
4	Learn of R&D advances	3	30

Asked to comment on the usefulness of the pharmaceutical industry's promotional activities the majority of the doctors indicated that their activities was of interest and of some use but not the main source of information (see Table 4).

Table 4. The Importance of Company Promotional Activities.

Category	No. of Doctors	%
Essential	9	6.21
Very useful	56	38.62
Some use	67	46.21
No use	13	8.97
Total	145	100.00

Doctors were then asked if they believed a brand name suggested an implicit guarantee of quality which 49% believed to be so. As 36% of all those surveyed preferred to prescribe brand drugs we looked at the reasons for such a preference, which in descending order of popularity were;

1. Company is better known and trusted
2. The quality of the product is better
3. The name is easier to distinguish
4. It is preferred by the patient
5. The efficacy of the product is better
6. The safety of the product is better
7. The consistency of the product
8. By prescribing brands you are supporting R&D

For those who did not prefer to prescribe brand products the most commonly indicated reason was the cost (38% indicated this), followed by the belief that generic and brand products were equivalent (15%).

AGE-RELATED DIFFERENCES IN PRESCRIBING INFLUENCES, SOURCES OF INFORMATION AND ATTITUDES TOWARDS PHARMACEUTICAL COMPANY PROMOTIONAL ACTIVITY

Prescribing Influences and Information Sources

Differences emerged when the surveyed doctors were divided into their two respective age-groups, those registered before 1980 and those registered in 1980 and afterwards.   Table 5 shows the various rankings of prescribing influences that emerged.   Although the top two influences, efficacy and previous personal experience, remained the same for both groups there were significant differences for some of the other factors specified.   In particular the importance of product price was quite different with the older doctor placing it fourth and 'quite important', while the 'younger' doctors ranked price sixth and as a 'useful, but not an important influence'.   Similarly the quality of a product, the spelling of a product name, the use of formularies and academic seminars all seem to be of more importance to the older doctor than to the younger.   The younger doctors seemed to list medical journals, colleagues experience, patient preference, company promotional information and external pressure of more influence in their prescribing decision.

Table 5. Factors of Influence for the two groups of doctors

	<1980				1980 > =		
Order	Factor	Rank	%	Order	Factor	Rank	%
1	Efficacy	5	78	1	Efficacy	5	80
2	Personal exp.	5	63	2	Personal exp.	5	70
3	Quality	5	41	3	Quality	4	48
4	Price	4	52	4	Medical Journals	4	62
5	Medical journals	4	59	5	Colleague exp.	4	46
6	Academic seminar	4	51	6	Price	3	38
7	Colleague exp.	4	44	7	Patient preference	4	44
8	Patient preference	3/4	34	8	Academic seminar	4	54
9	Formularies	4	32	9	Formularies	3	34
10	Quick recall	3	40	10	Quick recall	3	38
11	Promotional inf.	2	40	11	Promotional inf.	3	40
12	Spelling	1	46	12	External pressure	1	38
13	External pressure	1	41	13	Spelling	1	56

Differences were also found with reference to the sources of information specified (Table 6).   The older registered doctor put more emphasis on the academic seminars and conferences, formularies and company seminars as a useful source of information, while the younger doctors placed more emphasis on independent journals, patient feedback, colleagues experience, company sales representatives and company advertising in journals.

When looking at the general attitudes to prescribing and basic knowledge of the market inter-generational differences were also found.   The complicated generic spelling of drugs was a deterrent for a higher percentage of older generation (45% versus 40% of the younger doctors - Chi-square, $C^2=0.304$). More of the older doctors also thought a brand name suggested an implicit guarantee of quality (52% versus 44% of the younger doctors - $C^2=1.263$;). Despite all this, and perhaps surprisingly more of the younger doctors preferred to prescribe brand drugs (40% compared to 35% of the older doctors - $C^2=0.272$), and more of the older doctors made a decisive effort to prescribe all drugs by their generic form (39% compared to 36% - $C^2=0.12$). Using the Chi-square test to determine whether these differences were statistically significant at the 95% level with one degree of freedom ($C^2_{95}=$ 3.84) we found that they were not.

Table 6. Sources of Information for the two age groups

Order	Source of information (< 1980)	Rank	%	Order	Source of information (1980 > =)	Rank	%
1	Academic seminars	4	54	1	Independent journal	4	56
2	Independent journal	4	50	2	Patient feedback	4	64
3	Patient feedback	4	42	3 =	Academic seminars	4	48
4	Local drug inf.	4	41	3 =	Colleague exp.	4	44
5	Colleague exp.	4	46	5	Local drug inf.	4	32
6	Formularies	4	36	6	Company sales reps.	3	46
7	Company seminars	3	45	7	Formularies	3	34
8	Company sales reps	3	40	8	Company seminars	3	38
9	Company journal ad.	1	40	9	Company journal ad.	1/3	34
10	Company direct mail	1	47	10	Company direct mail	1	40

Fewer of the older doctors knew 'sometimes' of the dates of patent expiry (61% compared to 66% for the younger doctors) but again this was not a significant difference ($C^2=0.023$). In contrast a significant difference was found between the two groups in relation to awareness of generic entry into the market, with 52% of the older doctors 'sometimes' knowing about these dates compared to 72% of the younger generation — $C^2=5.798$.

Pharmaceutical Company Activity

26% of the older doctors saw a company sales representative once a month or less, with 8% never seeing a representative, while all the younger doctors saw a representative at least once a month. Similarly the average length of a visit by the sales representative was 10 minutes for the older doctors but 12.2 minutes for the younger doctor. Furthermore 38% of younger doctors thought company sales representatives successfully did their job, compared to 32% of the older doctors. Looking at the Chi-square statistic, $C^2=3.206$, this was a significant difference at the 90% level ($C^2_{90}=2.706$).

   Looking at the ranking of the types of information provided by companies 56% of the younger doctors found company promotional activities as quite important for learning about new products compared to 41% of the older doctors, a significant difference at the 90% level, $C^2=2.832$.   29% of the older doctors found this information quite important as a reminder of existing products compared to 24% of the younger doctors, although this was an insignificant difference, $C^2=0.022$. Meanwhile, 46% of the younger doctors found company promotional activities very useful compared to 35% of the older group, while 48% found it interesting and of some use compared to 45% of the older doctors. Neither of these differences were significant when tested. However the spread of the older doctors was interesting as it was much more varied. Over 9% categorising company promotional activity as essential compared to only 2% of the younger doctors but likewise almost 12% believed company activity to be a nuisance and a waste of resources compared to only 4% of the younger doctors.

CONCLUSIONS

Company promotional activity is not considered an important influence on the prescribing decision nor as a source of information by doctors. Perhaps the only concession they were prepared to admit was that the quick recall of a product name is useful, this being associated with the brand names. Nevertheless the responses given to various other questions imply that company promotion is effective. Obviously the most important use of the company promotional material is for learning about new products however this does not mean that such material is very influential. The fact that just under a half of all those surveyed believed that a brand name suggested an implicit guarantee of quality while 36% happily admitted to preferring brand name drugs when making their prescribing decisions suggests the effectiveness of company promotional campaigns. The reasons given for the brand preference also strengthen this conclusion. In particular the trust placed in the better known product and company itself, the belief that the quality of a brand drug was better and the ease with which the name could be distinguished all imply successful promotional campaigns. Other less important reasons were that of the efficacy, safety and consistency of the products which again indicated features which the company would promote heavily.

When one considers the fact that in 1991 pharmaceutical manufacturing spent $9bn on R&D but $10bn on marketing it's importance to the firm becomes obvious and it could be assumed that it must have some effect if so much money is committed to such expenditures (FDC Report 1991; Bleidt 1992).

In 1966 The Sainsbury Report declared sales representatives to be the prime source of information on new products (Holland 1977), while Winick 1980 found pharmaceutical sales representatives second only to professional journals as a source of reliable information on new drugs (Caudill 1992). Perhaps with the bad publicity concerning company marketing strategies doctors have become more cautious about the material and information given out or more reluctant to admit their reliance, maybe they simply do not realise the extent of influence such activity can have. In 1984 a DHSS draft circular on 'corruption' was sent out for consultation but was met with a response whereby few doctors accepted that they themselves were corrupted.

> Most believed they were quite untouched by the seductive ways of the industry's marketing men; that they were uninfluenced by the promotional propaganda they received; that they could enjoy a company's 'generosity' in the form of gifts and hospitality without prescribing its products. The harsh truth is that not one of us is impervious to the promotional activities of the industry and that the industry uses its various sales techniques because they are effective (Rawlins 1984:277).

Looking at another study conducted by Avorn *et al* (1982) two heavily marketed drugs whose pharmacological effects for common conditions were no better than over-the-counter (otc) preparations were considered. They discovered that those who prescribed these drugs tended to rely on industry sources of information yet they did not rank them as essentially important. A further study by Orlowski & Wateska (1992) found evidence that an expense-paid seminar at a resort was associated with a significant increases in the prescribing of the promoted drugs at one institution. They realised that this increase may be attributable to a realisation of the safety and efficacy of the promoted drugs however there was no noticeable change in the prescribing of those drugs it was designed to replace. The increased prescribing of this promoted drug was additional prescribing which illustrates the effectiveness of this means of promotional campaign.

> Physicians seem to perceive that their prescribing of drugs is influenced predominantly by scientific literature but in fact commercial sources of information such as advertising and interactions with detail personnel, play a major role.'
> (Orlowski & Wateska 1992:273)

Our finding that doctors rank company promotional activity as of little influence yet still maintain certain views which imply company influence corresponds with these findings.

When considering the different age-groups of the surveyed doctors some interesting differences were found in the percentage comparisons of various aspects of prescribing, however most of these proved insignificant when the Chi-square test was used. The main differences that did emerge as significant related to the awareness of generic entry onto the market, the use of information from companies and the competence of company sales representatives. The younger doctors proved more aware of generic entry onto the market, while significantly more of them found company promotional activity as a quite important source of information on new products. Finally significantly more younger doctors believed company sales representatives did their job properly.

With increased publicity over health care costs and governments efforts to encourage cost-effective prescribing it is perhaps not surprising that younger doctors were more aware of market conditions as no doubt their training has altered to take this into account With regards their belief that company material is quite important as a source of information of new products this may be characteristic of attempts to increase knowledge while experience is still limited. For these younger doctors medical journals, colleague experience, and patient preference were ranked higher in the list of prescribing influences, while for the sources of information more emphasis was placed on medical journals and patient feedback. These may imply a more active search for information by the younger, more inexperienced doctors.

Obviously methods of training will change over time which may account for some of the variations found, however there are other subtle differences in the order and rank of various sources of information. For example although both age-groups rank company sales representatives the same, the older doctors place it eighth as a source of information compared to sixth for the younger doctors. Perhaps in the search for more information the younger doctor is more open to all the material presented and less coloured by previous experiences and publicity. This implication may be reinforced by the fact significantly more of the younger doctors believed company sales representatives do their job properly (C^2=3.206, significant at the 90% level of significance).

Looking at the percentage figures obtained, more older doctors prescribed generically irrespective of availability, while price figured higher in the list of influences for their prescribing decision. It could be suggested that the older doctor feels the need to change prescribing attitudes and become more aware of pricing and generic competition, although no significant difference was found using the Chi-square test. Nevertheless considering those who preferred to prescribe generically significantly more older doctors indicating cost as a factor of influence which fits in with the above speculation (42% compared to 30% of the younger doctors which was significant at the 95% level, C^2=4.864).

Looking at the activity of companies in relation to the age-groups some further explanations may be derived. Firstly the younger doctor is visited more often and for longer than the older doctor. They are inexperienced in prescribing hence companies perhaps devote more time and energy on them to establish a relationship and help them form prescribing habits which will hopefully be beneficial for the company in the future. The older doctors will no doubt have already formed their opinions and habits from experience since registration, therefore the results from company attentiveness would not be as successful. It could be speculated that attitudes towards prescribing brand and generic products and pharmaceutical companies change with time.

REFERENCES

Avorn, Jerry; Chen, Milton; Hartley, Robert (1982) 'Scientific versus Commercial Sources of Influence on the Prescribing Behaviour of Physicians.' *American Journal of Medicine*, 72, July: 4 - 8.

Bleidt, Barry (1992) 'Recent Issues and Concerns about Pharmaceutical Industry Promotional Efforts.' *The Journal of Drug Issues*, 22 (2): 407 - 415.

Bradley, Colin P. (1992) 'Uncomfortable Prescribing Decisions: A Critical Incident Study.' *BMJ*, Vol. 304, 1 Feb.: 294 - 296

Caplow, Theodore; Raymond, John J. (1954) 'Factors Influencing the Selection of Pharmaceutical Products.' *Journal of Marketing*, 19/6:18 - 23

Caudill, T Shawn; Lurie, Nicole; Rich, Eugene C. (1992) 'The Influence of Pharmaceutical Industry Advertising on Physician Prescribing.' *The Journal of Drug Issues*, 22(2): 331 - 338.

Denig, P.; Haaijer-Ruskamp. F. M. (1992) 'Therapeutic Decision Making of Physicians.' *Pharmaceutisch Weekblad Scientific edition*, 14 (1):9 - 15

Goldfinger, Stephen E. (1990) 'Physicians and the Pharmaceutical Industry.' *Annals of Internal Medicine*, Vol. 112, No. 8:624 - 626

Hoffenberg, Raymond. (1986) 'The Relationship between Physicians and the Pharmaceutical Industry: A Report of the Royal College of Physicians.' *Journal of the Royal College of Physicians of London*, Vol. 20, No. 4:235 - 242

Holland, A. E. (1977) 'Representatives and Advertisement as Sources of Information.' *Postgraduate Medical Journal*, 53: 559 - 561.

Hurwitz, Mark A.; Caves, Richard E. (1988) 'Persuasion or Information? Promotion and the Shares of Brand-name and Generic Pharmaceuticals.' *Journal of Law and Economics*, 31 (2):299 - 320

Jennings, M. (1992) 'The Economics of Prescribing.' *Journal of the Royal College of Physicians of London*, Vol. 26, No. 1: 66 - 68.

Orlowski, James P.; Wateska, Leon. (1992) 'The Effects of Pharmaceutical Firm Enticements on Physician Prescribing Patterns; There's No Such Thing as a Free Lunch.' *CHEST*, 102(1), July:270 - 273

Rawlins, Michael D. (1984) 'Doctors and the Drug Makers' *The Lancet*, August 4: 276 - 278.

Smith, Mickey (1991) *'Pharmaceutical Marketing: Strategy and Cases.'* The Haworth Press Inc.

Stross, Jeoffrey K. (1987) 'Information Sources and Clinical Decisions.' *Journal of General Internal Medicines*, Pt. 2:155 - 159

APPENDIX — PRESCRIBING QUESTIONNAIRE

Date of medical registration:_____

Number of years at present practice:_____

Please circle or tick the appropriate answers (in some instances more than one answer may be appropriate therefore tick as many responses as required).

1. In general do you prefer to prescribe brand-name products **yes/no**

2. If you answered yes to the above the reason(s) for this preference is because; (tick as many responses as required)

    - the drug company is known and trusted
    - the quality is better
    - the efficacy is better
    - the safety is better
    - it is easier to distinguish by name

    Any other reasons: _____

    If the answer was no please state the reason(s)_____

3. Do you think a brand-name suggests "an implicit guarantee of quality"? (Reekie 1979) **yes/no**

4. Does the complicated generic spelling of drugs deter prescribing in an everyday clinic situation? **yes/no**

5. Are you aware of when the patent expires on brand-name drug? **yes/no/sometimes**

6. Are you aware of when generic equivalents enter the market? **yes/no/sometimes**

7. Do you make a decisive effort to prescribe all drugs by their generic name irrespective of their generic availability? **yes/no/sometimes**

8. What factors listed below influence your general prescribing and how important do you consider them to be on a scale of 1 - 5 as indicated below (please rank all the responses as appropriate)

    1 -- Of no importance/ influence
    2 -- Interesting but of no direct use
    3 -- Useful but not an important influence
    4 -- Quite important
    5 -- Very important

    - Previous personal experience of a product
    - Previous colleague experience of a product
    - Quality of a product
    - Efficacy of a product
    - Patient preference for a product

- Price of a product
- Spelling of a product name
- Quick recall of the product name
- Promotional information from drug companies
- External pressure - local health board
- academic seminars and conferences
- information read in medical journals
- formularies of the practice or local hospital
- Others: _____

9. Do you think visits by pharmaceutical company medical sales representatives
   serve their purpose as spreading relevant information on drugs   **yes/no/sometimes**

10. How often are you visited by a pharmaceutical company sales representative?

   - Once a week
   - Once a month
   - Other _____

How long do these visits tend to last?

   - 5 minutes
   - 10 minutes
   - 30 minutes
   - Other _____

11. Are there certain therapeutic drugs which are promoted more aggressively
    than others by the pharmaceutical companies   **yes/no**

   Suggestions: - Cardiovascular
                       - Anti-depressant
                       - Anti-ulcer
                       - Central nervous system
                       - Respiratory system
                       - Antibacterials
                       - Dermatologicals
                       - Musculoskeletal
                       - Genito-urinary/hormones
                       - Anti-cancers
                       - Others: _____

12. Are there any pharmaceutical companies who are significantly more
    aggressive in promoting their products than others?   **yes/no**

   Suggestions: - Merck
                       - Glaxo
                       - Bayer
                       - Hoechst
                       - SmithKline Beecham
                       - Wellcome
                       - Hoechst
                       - I.C.I.

- Roche
- Lilly
- Others:_____

13. Using the ranking system (1-5) from Question 7 how important would you say such
company promotional activity is as a source of information for the following:

- learning about new products
- reminders of existing products
- learning of new dosages, formulations & indications
- learning of advances made in R&D for future reference

14. Using the same ranking system as before circle the most appropriate number below to indicate
the importance you place on the following sources of information on products

- pharmaceutical company advertising in journals	1 2 3 4 5
- pharmaceutical company direct mailing	1 2 3 4 5
- pharmaceutical company seminars & conferences	1 2 3 4 5
- pharmaceutical company medical sales representatives	1 2 3 4 5
- academic seminars & conferences	1 2 3 4 5
- independent scientific journals	1 2 3 4 5
- local drug information services/hospital	1 2 3 4 5
- patient feedback on products	1 2 3 4 5
- colleague experiences with products	1 2 3 4 5
- formularies in local practice/hospital	1 2 3 4 5

15. From the following how would you categorise pharmaceutical company promotional activities?
(tick as appropriate)

- an extremely useful and essential source of information
- a very useful source of information but not the main one
- interesting and of some use but mainly rely on training
- of no use and mainly a nuisance, a waste of resources
- other: _____

Any other general comments would be much appreciated on any of the above questions or
on other points you feel to be relevant.

8 Pharmacy Policy and Practice — The Future

ALAN HAYCOX

University of Keele

INTRODUCTION

Since the inception of the NHS in 1948 the British health care system has been dominated by two influences — one driven by economics and the other by science and technology. The first influence is that of resource scarcity with the pressure to contain costs emanating primarily from the government. The second influence is derived from the exponential rate of progress in developing and improving treatment modalities within the health care system. Nowhere within the health care system is this pressure felt more acutely than within the pharmaceutical sector. The NHS is being continuously bombarded with new developments in diagnosis and treatment many of which crept into clinical practice without any formal evaluation of their comparative value in relation to other potential developments. Such "creeping development" was normally supported merely as a consequence of the power exercised (or noise level generated) by the clinical champions of the innovation. At times of real resource growth the implications of such sub-optimal decision making were less evident given that the need to confront powerful clinical pressure groups was less obvious when financial discipline was not as stringent. However the removal of resource slack from the NHS has required managers to become more rigorous in evaluating and choosing between service options.

The primary aim of this paper is to examine the fundamental changes that have taken place within the British National Health Service and to analyse their implications for the evaluation and utilization of pharmaceutical products. The initial hypothesis is that the information requirements of the new NHS have significantly changed and are not being adequately met by current sources of pharmaceutical evaluation. The nature and implications of the NHS reforms for pharmaceutical evaluation have been fully discussed elsewhere (St Leger *et al* 1992) but in essence the changes separate purchasing from the provision of health care services by the creation of an internal market. The key role of the newly developed purchasing teams is to assess the health needs of their populations and to structure their

Managerial Issues in the Reformed NHS. Edited by M.Malek, P.Vacani, J.Rasquinha & P.Davey
© 1993 John Wiley & Sons Ltd

purchasing decisions so as to maximize the health gain derived from a given budget. In order to achieve such an aim requires detailed and accurate information concerning the comparative costs and benefits of each available service provision option. Unfortunately the formal structure underlying the evaluation of new pharmaceutical products does not produce the type of information required by purchasers in making such decisions. This paper suggests ways in which the focus of such evaluations can be widened to reflect the enhanced information needs of NHS policy makers.

THE CHANGING MARKET PLACE — THE ROLE AND OBJECTIVES OF THE NEW NHS

The current relationship between purchasers and providers within the reformed NHS is in a state of flux. Certain purchasing agencies are beginning to ask more fundamental questions with regard to the structure, quality and quantity of services received by their residents. They are beginning to take seriously their role as the "champion of the people" despite the fact that health care providers who have been silently championing patients since 1948 may feel a little aggrieved at the apparent belittlement of their role in the health care system.

The bewildering speed at which the NHS reforms have been implemented has been severely criticised even by proponents of the reforms. However it must be recognised that all organisations must change and adapt otherwise they will inevitably suffer in the face of an ever changing operational environment. The bigger the organisation the greater the problems inherent in any attempt to introduce a dynamic element that allows it to adapt to new demands and modes of operation. Such change inevitably imposes costs during the transition as staff within the organisation become aware of, and adjust, to the new demands and expectations placed upon them. In such circumstances a policy of fundamental change (rather than gradual evolution) within any organisation should only be undertaken where the benefits derived (better fulfilment of organisational objectives) are expected to be greater then the costs incurred (disruption of the organisation) during the transitional period.

The vast scale of operation implies that the problems of fundamental change in the NHS will inevitably be enormous, but so too may be the subsequent benefits. The impact of such changes should be analysed in relation to the extent to which they facilitate the long term achievement of NHS organisational objectives. A simple dichotomy of objectives will suffice for the purpose of this paper:

1. Equal access to people of equal need The *accessibility* objective of the NHS.
2. Maximising health care provision within a given resource constraint —
   the *efficiency* objective of the NHS.

The use of such broad objectives introduce many semantic problems (what do we mean by access, need, health care and resources?) but any discussion of change that does not focus upon organisational objectives will prove to be essentially barren. Therefore it is necessary to analyse the extent to which the practical objectives of the NHS, with regard to pharmaceutical policy and practice, have been fundamentally altered by the NHS reforms.

THE AIMS OF PHARMACEUTICAL POLICY AND PRACTICE

There exists an inevitable tension between the pharmaceutical industry and the Health Service. Pharmaceutical companies are not charitable institutions but consist of competitive businesses whose primary focus is, quite correctly, upon the quality of their balance sheet. In many ways they represent a good role model for the NHS given the frequent exhortation to improve the business orientation of NHS managers. In the past the pharmaceutical industry displayed great prowess in taking advantage of lax or non-existent NHS pharmaceutical planning procedures. Such an observation does not represent a criticism given that the pharmaceutical industry simply responded efficiently to the system imposed upon it by the NHS.

The fundamental need is for the NHS to alter the incentive structure facing the pharmaceutical industry in order to ensure co-terminosity between the aims of both the industry and the NHS. In theory such co-terminosity is simple to achieve. The pharmaceutical industry aims to maximize profits while the NHS aims to maximise health gain therefore all that is required is to ensure that innovative, resource saving drugs offering the greatest health gain are recognized and supported by the NHS and provide the greatest level of profitability to the pharmaceutical industry. In times of resource scarcity all companies become increasingly responsive to market signals and the NHS as market maker has the power to alter the structure of incentives facing the pharmaceutical industry to the benefit of both parties.

> "In times of restraint it is to the pharmaceutical industry's benefit that there be clearer and more rational procedures by which innovation is taken on by the NHS. In the absence of these procedures, products which provide significant benefit to patients, which are clearly innovative and which may save resources, may not be supported. A market place with haphazard and changeable rules works to nobody's benefit."
> (St Leger *et al* 1992:307).

There is an ever present tendency within the NHS to denigrate the pharmaceutical industry for its "unethical" policies. However, such criticism fundamentally misconstrues the nature of the relationship between the industry and the NHS. The pharmaceutical industry may provide the engine room but it is the policy makers within the NHS that are steering the pharmaceutical ship. If we attempt to construct pharmaceutical policy and practice on an inadequate information base then our pharmaceutical ship is inevitably heading for the rocks. In such circumstances it seems a little churlish to blame an efficient engine room whose only contribution is to land us on the rocks a little more quickly than perhaps we had anticipated.

Rationality in NHS pharmaceutical policy requires effected and concerted management action in at least five areas:

- **Pharmaceutical planning** — Accurate identification of current and future needs for pharmaceutical products.
- **Pharmaceutical rationing** — ensuring the rigorous evaluation of pharmaceutical products to ensure that maximum health gain is derived within the level of resources available.
- **Pharmaceutical resources** — Rigorous evaluation should emphasize the extent to which potential health gains in this area are not being realised as a consequence of resource shortages. In addition future resource planning in this area must take account of the impact of such factors as demographic changes (an increasingly elderly population), policy changes (an increased emphasis on case finding) and pharmaceutical innovation (drugs being developed to confront diseases that were not previously amenable to pharmaceutical intervention).
- **Consumerism in pharmaceutical policy** — ensuring that the public are informed about the direction and priorities of pharmaceutical policy and constructing an effective and ongoing mechanism by which consumer views are effectively identified and acted upon.
- **Monitoring** — Implementation of a mechanism to ensure that the previous management aims are being achieved.

Each of these five management tasks, are interdependent and the under fulfilment of one task would almost inevitably adversely affect the achievement of the other tasks. For example, the rational allocation of health care resources, inevitably relies upon effective planning and effective rationing. The emphasis in each of these areas must be on collaboration with the pharmaceutical industry to ensure the required co-terminosity of aims and the provision of an appropriate incentive structure to which the industry can respond in an appropriate manner.

A COLLABORATIVE STRUCTURE FOR PHARMACEUTICAL POLICY

Pharmaceutical Planning

The NHS has always in the past primarily taken a reactive role to the direction of research and innovation by the pharmaceutical industry. The normal procedure was to wait until drugs had been developed and licensed prior to addressing issues relating to their utilization and targeting. A more mutually beneficial approach would be for the NHS to work with the industry identifying crucial areas of need that could be ameliorated by pharmaceutical innovation. In this manner NHS policy makers could assist in targeting the research and development efforts of the pharmaceutical industry. Equally a more proactive relationship with the NHS should assist the pharmaceutical industry in choosing which of the many potentially beneficial compounds developed by their scientists holds the greatest potential in the marketplace.

Pharmaceutical innovation represents a lengthy and inexact process and the price of failure (bringing a drug to the marketplace only to find that it is not successful) is inevitably high. As such any process that facilitates customers and suppliers to work together in identifying the main elements of current and future needs for pharmaceutical products must surely be of value to both parties.

Pharmaceutical Rationing

Broken down to its crudest level the role of the NHS is to contribute additional value to its patients. The NHS applies appropriate inputs (labour, land capital and entrepreneurship) into a production process (an operation or some other form of intervention) that results in an output (normally in terms of the improved health status of the patient). The transformation process undertaken in the hospital adds value to the recipient (the patient) by improving the patients' health condition, hopefully sufficiently to allow discharge from the hospital environment. The value of the transformation process depends upon two factors.

- The overall extent and nature of the patients improvement in health status.
- How this production of health compares with the natural progression of the disease.

The application of such a model to evaluating the value added by pharmaceutical products is complicated by two fundamental difficulties...

- Drugs are normally used simply as part of the treatment regime and in any such areas of joint production it is difficult to isolate the specific output derived from any individual input.
- The measure of patient benefit (health gain) is beset by philosophical and practical difficulties.

It is to the benefit of all participants within the health system to ensure that we are utilizing the current stock of resources is utilised in the optimal manner. Only in this way can an effective case be made for additional resources to be provided that will allow us to obtain further health gains from pharmaceutical products. The key to illustrating the further health gains that could be obtained from marginal increments in resource availability is the rigorous and comprehensive evaluation of pharmaceutical products. The manner in which the pharmaceutical industry and the NHS can address these issues in a collaborative manner is examined below.

THE COLLABORATIVE EVALUATION OF PHARMACEUTICAL PRODUCTS

It is no longer sufficient for a pharmaceutical product to simply show that it is safe and provides patient benefit. In order to make rational decisions it is necessary to further assess:
- *How much* benefit does the product provide and to which target groups?
- At what *cost* is this patient benefit obtained?

The concept of opportunity cost is at the centre of economic analysis in this area. The ideal would be to be able to afford all drugs that could possibly provide benefit to patients but this is not a realistic possibility. Unfortunately the methodology underlying clinical trials is focused primarily upon addressing biologically orientated issues that fall within the realm of clinical procedures. In cancer studies survival curves are calculated together with estimates of the size of the primary tumour and hence such factors become the sole clinical determinant of the relative success or failure of a new pharmaceutical product. Unfortunately such clinically relevant measures of success may bear little relation to the factors that are deemed to be important by the patient and patients family. Issues of quality of life and the perception of being in control of their lives may be of greater importance to patients than the mere prolongation of life at any cost in terms of human dignity and suffering. In extreme cases patients may withdraw from treatment in order to enforce *their* comparative valuation of short term life quality in relation to long term gains in their quantity of life. The development of a range of credible measuring instruments (Jaeschke et al 1992, McDowell and Newell 1987) for quality of life studies facilitates their routine but sensitive incorporation into a more comprehensive evaluation of pharmaceutical products.

The extent and nature of clinical and quality of life changes are necessary but not sufficient elements in pharmaceutical evaluation. A comprehensive pharmaceutical evaluation should not remain the exclusive domain of clinicians and statisticians but requires collaboration with psychologists, sociologists, information scientists, health economists and other health professionals . As the nature of new pharmaceutical products becomes more complex so too does the range of skills required for their effective evaluation. Economic and quality of life analyses need to be incorporated as an integral component of any evaluation and not merely tagged on as a marketing strategy after the real clinical trial has been undertaken. This requires a fundamental shift in the ethos, orientation and design of clinical trials in order to meet the new information needs of NHS decision makers. The objective of the analysis is no longer just to show that any product is relatively safe and provides clinical benefit, but rather to specify how much benefit is provided, in what form the benefits occur, and how such benefits relate to the patients' overall quality of life. Equally the analysis should address a range of complex issues relating to the level of resources consumed in utilizing new drugs and level of the opportunity cost incurred. The following sections analyse the extent to which current clinical trials properly augmented provide an adequate structure for obtaining this more comprehensive and valuable dataset.

IMPLICATIONS FOR PHARMACEUTICAL TRIALS

The clinical evaluation of pharmaceutical products attempts to evaluate their efficacy and safety utilizing scientific research principles and employing a rigorous code of ethics. The organization and analysis of such trials represents an amalgamation of medicine with statistics and requires close collaboration between the pharmaceutical industry and the medical profession. The organization and structure of such studies are rigorously controlled and must follow a set pattern:

Phase I Studies

At this stage a new compound has been developed but its characteristics (toxicity, dose tolerance, general pharmacological properties, possible therapeutic effects and potential interactions with other compounds) are largely unknown and hence there is a natural and quite appropriate reluctance to experiment on man. Regulatory authorities insist on extensive animal testing despite the fact that there is frequently a tenuous relationship between the effects of drugs in animals and those in man. As such, having gained an indication of the impact of a drug with animal experimentation, healthy adult male human volunteers become the final experimental animal. Given the uncertainty of the drugs' impact in humans, early trials should be cautious and utilize very low doses. The first administration of drugs to man should take place in a specialized unit devoted to such studies and with ready access to a range of specialized medical facilities. Such studies commence with single rising doses initially at between 1-2% of the maximum tolerated dose in animals and with no increase in dosage until the results of the previous groups safety tests are known.

The aim of such studies is to predict a safe dose level for utilization in stage II studies. Only once single dose administration has been successfully completed can multiple dose studies commence. The drug, or placebo, is provided for a period of normally 14 days to examine the extent of a cumulative toxicity. Typically 6 groups of 8 volunteers (5 with the drug 3 with placebo) are analysed with the results of each group being analysed sequentially prior to the next group having the drug administered. The main focus of phase I studies are to examine the pharmacological impact of the drug in man and examine the maximum tolerated single or multiple doses that are commensurate with a drugs safety. Phase II studies take the well tolerated doses developed in phase I that provide sufficient patient benefit to warrant further investigation and analysis.

Phase II Studies

At this stage the drug is applied to patients as opposed to healthy volunteers with the aim of confirming the safety information obtained in Phase I and developing information concerning the efficacy of the drug. The calculation of the therapeutic ratio (safety compared to efficacy) provides the first indication of the potential value of any new drug in the marketplace. Relatively small numbers of patients are monitored in detail in comparison with placebo or alternative drug therapy depending on the condition being treated. The number of patients required for

Phase II trials depends on the comparative advantage of the new drug over existing compounds and the statistician should ensure that sufficient patients are incorporated into the trial to show a statistically significant difference between the new drug and existing therapy. Phase II trials tend to be of short duration and frequently throw up results that are indicative rather than conclusive . As such the decision to continue from phase II trials is frequently based upon clinical and pharmacological judgement rather than the statistically proven value of the compound. In such cases issues relating to the level and impact of side effects, the level of cumulative toxicity and the comparative efficacy of the treatment need to be weighed.

For the first time, however, we have crossed the rubicon and entered the world of the health economist. A range of economic issues should be considered at this stage when considering the potential cost effectiveness of developing the drug. For example how big is the potential market for the drug? Is the cost of treatment with this drug likely to be competitive in comparison to existing and potential competitors? Such questions require the drug company to sensitively weigh the marginal potential benefits that are expected to be derived from the drugs' development with the marginal additional costs incurred in getting the drug to the marketplace. As such analysis of phase II trials inevitably require a mixture of clinical and economic judgements prior to deciding to proceed to stage III.

Phase III Studies

At this stage the aim is to establish the comparative safety and efficacy of a drug with a view to discerning the optimum method of future treatment for the target group of patients. By this stage all trials should be utilizing the anticipated final formulation. Phase III trials require a great deal of time, effort and money from the pharmaceutical company and should only be embarked upon if they are convinced that the potential future benefits exceed the significant costs incurred during this stage of the drug costing process. The possibility of large profits can be enticing, but the company also needs to remember the large number of newly developed drugs that have emphasised the ease with which it is possible to make substantial losses. It is tempting to focus on the costs already incurred as a reason to continue, but past costs become irrelevant to effective current decision making. The balance of potential costs and benefits for the new drug is likely to be continuously changing over its development and requires detailed and frequent skilled assessment.

Double blind randomised control trials are commonly accepted as being the best method of evaluating new drugs. Patients are randomly assigned to the new treatment or the standard existing treatment to establish the comparative effectiveness and safety of the new drug in comparison to current practice . Given that the trial is analysing the marginal improvements over current therapy much larger patient numbers will be required to achieve statistically significant results. The aim is to analyze the smallest number of patients commensurate with the need to obtain statistical significance in the results obtained. Statistical monitoring can employ closed sequential designs such that once a predetermined level of significance has been reached the trial can be stopped.

The focus in phase III trials is almost entirely on obtaining statistically significant evidence concerning comparative clinical efficacy and safety. This is done by expanding the quantity of patients clinically evaluated until the statistician cries 'enough'. Surely there is another way? One that expands the *quality* of the dataset obtained rather than continuously expanding the number of patients contained in the trial.

Many new compounds offer relatively minor therapeutic advantages and hence may find their usage difficult to justify on the basis of a purely clinical trial. Such minor clinical advantages (reduced nausea and hair loss in oncological treatment) may be of enormous value to the patient in maintaining their quality of life during treatment and helping to ensure a reduced drop out rate and increased compliance with treatment. Such impacts will not be adequately picked up unless the stage III trial is broadened to include a detailed assessment of the impact of the drug upon patient quality of life - a much wider concept not currently utilized in the majority of phase III studies. The inclusion of quality of life studies argues for a widening rather than a deepening of phase III studies in order to ascertain drug impacts that are of importance and relevance to the patient themselves. In such circumstances statistical significance would not depend upon expanding the number of possibly inappropriate measurements undertaken but rather it would be dependent on measuring a wider range of appropriate changes in a smaller patient population. Such an approach would also have the important ethical advantage of not exposing excessive numbers of patients unnecessarily to what remains a relatively untried treatment regime.

Phase IV Studies and Post Marketing Surveillance

Stage IV studies and post marketing surveillance focuses on the impact of the drug after it has become generally available. The rarefied world of double blind randomised control trials focusing in a controlled manner on well defined target groups has been left behind and replaced by the real world prescribing habits of physicians and the real world compliance and inexactitudes of patients.

Ideally phase IV studies should consist of prospective clinical trials obtaining a large amount of comparative patient information concerning the impact of a drug in practice. All of the less scientific monitoring activities are normally included under the description of post marketing surveillance. Varying responses to the drug may become apparent in different age groups and in patients with different co-morbidities that may have been excluded from analysis in earlier phases. Equally new indications may appear as may new contraindications and drug interactions that will all add new information to the drug profile.

Phase IV studies provide evidence of the actual marginal costs and benefits of a new drug in comparison to established drugs and hence add further to the data that could be utilized in a comprehensive economic analysis of the drug. The results of such an analysis would help in ascertaining whether the price, targeting and marketing focus of the drug is optimal given its use and value in the marketplace. It has previously been argued (Dollery, 1976) that phase IV studies should focus on ways of making drugs more effective and it is only one minor step from this recommendation to emphasising the need to focus upon the cost-effectiveness of new drugs as used in practice.

Post marketing surveillance should be undertaken for all drugs given the ever present possibility of complications arising as a consequence of medium to long term exposure to drug therapy. At this stage economic and social aspects may begin to be incorporated into the marketing strategy for the drug. The actual cost-effectiveness of any drug can only be assessed after the drug has been marketed because the impact of the drug has to be demonstrated in a large number of patients in significantly different environments. Equally the targeting of the drug will effectively determine its cost effectiveness given that the more closely it concentrates on patients who are likely to receive the greatest benefit then the higher will be its actual cost effectiveness. Conversely the more widely focused the drugs' target group (inevitably mixing patients receiving major benefit with patients receiving little or no benefit) then the lower will be the measured cost effectiveness of the drug in the real world prescribing situation. The potential value of a comprehensive stock of such information to purchasing agencies struggling to make optimal use of an inadequate drug budget cannot be overemphasised.

CONCLUSION

The ethos of the NHS has fundamentally altered with purchasing developing detailed business plans that require providers to justify the cost effectiveness of new pharmaceutical innovations. Suppliers of health care are becoming increasingly aware that their long term viability can only be ensured by the provision of services that are demanded by purchasers. In order to justify the utilization of new pharmaceutical products physicians thus require information not only on the safety and efficacy but also on the cost effectiveness of new pharmaceutical products.

The ability of society to confront disease and infirmity is continuously being expanded as a consequence of the efforts of the pharmaceutical industry. The potential health gains to patients that arise from such developments are likely to prove to be enormous. In order to capitalise upon such potential benefits the NHS requires effective planning and rigorous evaluation to target its use of resources in this area. Such effective use of existing resources will allow the NHS to put forward a more effective case for new resources to be able to capitalize on the high marginal benefits arising from pharmaceutical products that otherwise could not be afforded. The failure to ensure an adequate response from the NHS inevitably leads to sub optimal performance given that pharmaceutical resources become overwhelmed by the demands made upon it. Ad hoc 'coping strategies' become necessary which are sub-optimal both from the perspective of the organisation and in the view of society as a whole.

A range of additional problems arise for managers operating in the NHS that result from the fact that they merely control one part of the overall system that determines the health or their consumers. A range of factors significantly affecting health will inevitably arise as a consequence of actions that occur outside the control of managers within the health service itself. Changes in the economic system will inevitably feed through to the health system, in a number of ways. An increase in unemployment locally, will lead, to an increase in physical and psychological morbidity, leading to an increased level of demand for pharmaceutical resources. Equally, the level and distribution of disposable income will significantly affect the level of health needs, and hence, the demands placed upon pharmaceutical resources.

The health of the national economy will also be a fundamental determinal of the availability of resources to the NHS and hence to the pharmaceutical budget. We can assist our case for more resources by showing that we utilize our current resources in an optimal manner. This requires us to demonstrate that we are maximizing the health gain that is derived from the current drug stock and have initiated a rigorous evaluative structure to determine the value-for-money obtained from the flow of new pharmaceutical products. In order to rectify this situation and ensure that pharmaceutical innovations that provide the greatest health gain are supported it is necessary to ensure that new products are subject to comprehensive and timely clinical and economic scrutiny prior to their launch and dissemination within the health care system. Such a policy requires a common, structured and agreed approach to the evaluation of new pharmaceutical agents. In order to achieve this it is necessary for the NHS and pharmaceutical industry to collaborate closely in constructing an information system that addresses broader questions than those currently addressed by the structure of clinical evaluation. Both the NHS and the pharmaceutical industry need to ensure that evaluative studies rigorously address issues that effectively inform the process of policy making within the NHS. The fundamental changes within the NHS emphasize the need for a broader range of questions to be addressed by pharmacological evaluation, in order to capitalize on the enormous potential benefits that could occur as a consequence of the changes to both the NHS and the pharmaceutical industry.

REFERENCES

Dollery C. T. (1976) The assessment of efficacy toxicity and quality of care in long-term drug treatment. Walstenholme, G. O'Connor. M (eds) Research and Medical Practice: Their interaction, Ciba Foundation Symposium 44, American Elsevier, 73-88.

Jaeschke. R. *et al* (1992) Quality of life instruments in the evaluation of need drugs, pharmacoeconomics, 1, 84-94.

McDowell I and Newell, C (1987) measuring health - a guide to rating scales and questionnaires. Oxford University press, New York.

Mugglestone, C.J. (1986) Phase II and Phase III Studies, Glenny, H and Nelmes, P (eds) Handbook of clinical drug research, Blackwell scientific publications, Oxford. 94-126.

Rogers H. J and Spector R. G. (1986) Phase I studies, Glenny, H and Nelmes P (eds) op. cit. 33-58.

Stevens, E. A. (1986) Phase IV and Post Marketing Surveillance, Glenny, H. and Nelmes, P. (eds) op. cit. 127-150.

St. Leger, S. *et al* (1992) Evaluation of Pharmaceutical innovation. Pharmacoeconomics, 1, 306-311.

9 The Role of the Dental Health Service Consumer in Strategic Decision Making

DOUGLAS EADIE[1], AMANDA HAYWOOD[1], LILA PAVI[2] & ELIZABETH KAY[2]

[1]University of Strathclyde
[2]University of Glasgow

INTRODUCTION

It is well documented that Scotland has a comparatively poor dental health record (Todd 1982 & 1983), particularly among young children in the West of Scotland (Pitts and Davies 1988). Some advances have however been made in the up-take of preventive services and dental screening but these advances have been mainly with more affluent middle class groups. As a result the differences in oral health standards between those living in deprived areas and those living in less disadvantaged areas has become increasingly wide (Todd 1982 & 1983).

This problem has been acknowledged at policy level (HMSO 1979 & 1986) but it was considered important that initiatives designed to combat the problem be preceded by research. Hence in 1989 the Chief Scientists Office in Scotland commissioned this study to identify the possible barriers to the up-take of these preventive services amongst those living in deprived areas and to provide guidance upon how these barriers might be broken down.

METHOD

The study as a whole started in late 1989 and ran for some two and a half years. The main feature of the study was to draw direct comparisons between adults living in deprived inner city housing schemes and adults living in more affluent suburbs. The comparisons were made using three sets of measures illustrated below in figure 1.

The main element of the research involved conducting interview based research with two sub-samples of deprived and affluent groups. This involved assessing levels of knowledge for issues such as availability of preventive services as well as taking

Managerial Issues in the Reformed NHS. Edited by M.Malek, P.Vacani, J.Rasquinha & P.Davey
© 1993 John Wiley & Sons Ltd

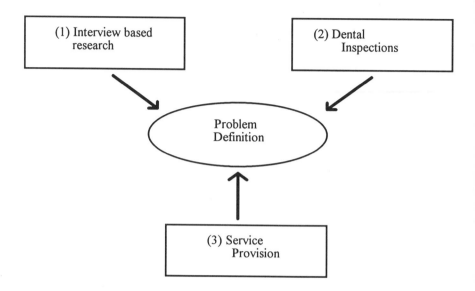

Figure 1. Methods of comparison

measures of attitude towards the services and in what circumstances the services were actually being used.

The interview element of the study was split into two stages. Given that previous studies in this area have been only partially successful in identifying the barriers to the use of dental screening (Williams, 1972; Weirs, 1980; and Wallstron, 1978) it was decided that in order to provide new insights and establish more fruitful lines of enquiry, to first of all use an open-ended exploratory research procedure. Hence, the first stage of interviewing involved using qualitative focus groups.

This involved running a series of six informal focus groups each made up of eight residents from the areas under investigation and run by a professional group moderator. The respondents were recruited from the different communities by professional market research interviewers and the groups were conducted in local community halls and centres. The discussions themselves ran for about one to one and a half hours were recorded on audio tape and then later transcribed for content analysis. The results from this initial exploratory stage were then used to aid the design of a structured questionnaire.

The second stage of the research involved administering this questionnaire on a face-to-face basis with a sample of some 850 respondents, drawn at random from residents of both the deprived and more affluent areas. The main aim of this second stage of research was to quantify and validate the findings of the group discussion research.

In addition to being interviewed, participants were also given the opportunity to have a dental inspection or check-up. This data allowed the research to assess the oral health status of the two sub-samples through the measurement of numbers of missing, filled and decaying teeth. It also enabled the research to assess respondents' treatment needs in terms of corrective treatment required, the preservation of decayed teeth and the need for dentures and dental plates.

Finally, the research also made an objective assessment of the levels of service provision in the areas in which the sub-samples were drawn. This assessed service accessibility by measuring the mean distance to the nearest surgery from participants homes and also service availability by measuring, amongst other things mean waiting times, dentist to patient ratios and the use of recall systems, i.e. whether and how patients were invited along for dental check-ups.

RESULTS

The key findings to emerge from the initial exploratory phase of the research are summarised below. The qualitative findings confirmed that those people from deprived areas were less likely to attend their dentist and that those from more affluent areas were more likely to attend for dental check-ups. The research then sought to explain the reasons for these different levels of attendance. The subsequent findings were wide ranging but two particular lines of enquiry proved fruitful in helping to explain the different attendance levels.

Firstly, the research focused specifically upon preventive services posing the question - were there any perceived differences in the quality of the preventive services offered? It then broadened out its frame of reference to look at dental services in general and asked the question - were there any differences in the types of dental service they wanted?

The differing results from these two different lines of enquiry proved very revealing.

Quality of Preventive Services

Six quality factors were examined using the discussion groups:

- **information requests** — awareness of preventative services and their importance to dental health,
- **service availability** — whether or not respondents knew of a dental practice they could attend for these services,
- **accessibility** — how easy it was to get to the nearest dental practice in terms of travel distance, transport and opening times,
- **service cost** — perceived value for money of the preventative services offered,
- **image** — of the dental profession as a whole,
- **service environment** — how well were the services being delivered, how friendly, approachable and helpful were the dental staff and how amenable was the surgery atmosphere to ensuring customer satisfaction?

The findings from each area are described in turn:

Information
All respondents who took part in the study knew of the existence of preventive services and were aware that regular attendance was important to good dental health. Failure to use the services was not therefore due to ignorance or any lack of knowledge.

Availability
Similarly, many respondents were already registered with a dentist and all of them knew of a dental practice they could attend for treatment. There were therefore few problems with availability.

Accessibility
With regards accessibility few respondents reported any problems in obtaining access to their dentist. The proximity of the dental surgery did not therefore emerge as an importance factor either.

Cost
The issue of cost and value for money initially seemed to represent an important factor in uptake, but some important differences arose with many non-attenders from the deprived sub-sample claiming that dental check-ups were too expensive. However, more detailed questioning revealed that those making these claims were not aware of the charges involved, were unaware of whether or not they were eligible for free treatment and most revealing of all, many of these people had not attended for check-ups in the past even when they were known to be available free of charge on the National Health Service.

This suggested that cost, rather than being an important influence on levels of attendance was instead being used to rationalise non-attendance and that other more fundamental factors were responsible for the low attendance levels.

Image
With the professions image, those living in the more deprived areas had less confidence in the dental profession than their less disadvantaged counter-parts.

There was a tendency amongst those living in the deprived areas to take the view that attending the dentist 'when there was nothing wrong with your teeth' (i.e. when you were not in any pain or discomfort) was 'asking for trouble.' It was widely believed that when attending for a check-up 'nine times out of ten' your dentist would find something wrong which required follow-up treatment. Many were sceptical of the dentists motives and claimed that it was in the dentists interests to find problems.

The research was not in a position to validate these claims but it was clear that the direct link between treatment and payment (i.e. paying on the premises) did leave the profession open to this kind of criticism.

Service environment

Poor service environment was the reason most commonly given for opting not to attend for dental check-ups largely because it was responsible for arousing considerable fear and anxiety

A number of important barriers emerged here. For example, building up the confidence to make an appointment for many often involved considerable courage. It was not uncommon for people to have to make several attempts before they were able to go to the dentist. Waiting in the surgery waiting area was also responsible for creating anxiety. This was often described as having a very tense atmosphere. The actual treatment itself was often found to be unpleasant; the loss of control experienced when lying on the dentists chair, the invasion of the mouth and unfamiliar and alien smells, sounds, bright lights and equipment all contributed to these unpleasant feelings.

Importantly, though, those from the more affluent areas were just as likely to relate these kinds of fears and anxieties as those from the deprived areas. The only difference to emerge here was that those from the deprived communities tended to display higher levels of fear. They often told chilling stories of how they had been treated by dentists during their childhood and how school dentists in Glasgow at that time were actually thought to 'enjoy inflicting pain on their patients.'

Overall, then, there were very few differences in the perceived quality of the services between the two sample groups that explained the differing attendance levels. The second line of enquiry, were there any differences in the type of dental services they were looking for, provided more fruitful in explaining these differences.

Types of Dental Service Wanted

Here the questioning procedure was broadened out beyond respondents knowledge and experience of preventive services to establish what dental services they felt best suited their needs and priorities. The aim here was to gain a consumers eye-view of the role and importance of dental health and dental services in their lives.

The perceived needs and wants of the two sub-samples differed quite dramatically. Those from the more affluent, less deprived backgrounds tended to attach particular importance to having and keeping their teeth and upon good dental health and despite the fears they often had about attending the dentist they welcomed regular reminders from the dentist to attend for dental check-ups.

Those from the more disadvantaged groups on the other hand although they recognised the importance of regular check-ups to dental health and although they often encouraged their own children to attend for such check-ups they themselves tended to place far less emphasis on having good teeth. They instead tended to attach more importance to treatment orientated services and in particular to emergency treatment services. For them the main role for the dental professional was to offer help in alleviating suffering. Hence they wanted fast and efficient pain relief services. They did not want to get involved in extended courses of treatment nor to have to attend for regular dental check-ups.

These findings couple with those described previously suggested that the reason why those living in more deprived communities opt not to take up preventive services is far less to do with any disparity in the actual delivery or quality of the services on offer, and far more to do with differences in the actual values that the groups placed on their teeth and on oral health standards in general.

These differing values were further expressed in the group discussions in a number of ways; though differences in their oral health expectations, through their preparedness to talk about their teeth and through the images they associated with the type of people who regularly attend for check-ups.

With regards to oral health expectations, those from the more deprived communities were often more happy to accept that loosing teeth was part and parcel of growing old. Indeed some took the view that having teeth removed brought to an end a lot of worry and pain. For this reason it was not uncommon for extractions to be preferred to preservation treatment. It was also noticeable that the wearing of dentures and dental plates was more of a norm in these communities. Those from more affluent backgrounds on the other hand were far more likely to adopt the alternative view, wishing instead to retain their natural teeth for as long as possible and opting for treatment that helped preserve their teeth.

There was also a much greater degree of openness amongst those from the more deprived areas when discussing their teeth. For example in one instance, when discussing dental plates a member of the discussion group removed his dental plate to show other members what it looked like and how it fitted. In contrast, those from more affluent communities taking part in the discussion groups were observably more restrained in their comments and more reluctant to volunteer information about their oral health status to other members of the group particularly on the subject of denture wearing.

These different values were also reflected in the images associated with the wearing of dentures and attendance for dental check-ups. For example, those from the more affluent or non-deprived communities associated denture wearing with negative images of ageing and poor social up-bringing while those from the deprived communities were more likely to describe someone who looked after their teeth and who regularly attended for dental check-ups as someone who was 'well-off' and importantly, as someone who was not from 'their side of town.'

These findings clearly illustrate how oral health status and the use of dental services have broader social meanings which go beyond that of physical health and well being. These differences are typified by these two contrasting comments made during the discussion. The first, from a resident of Castlemilk, a deprived inner city housing scheme in Glasgow and the second from someone from a more affluent Glasgow suburb.

> "(Natural teeth) .... aren't something that's going to cost you your life. The worst you
> can do is lose them and then you'd just get false ones. It's not that important to you."
> (Deprived)

"I would like to have them (natural teeth) until the day I die. I would hate to have false teeth .... It's the thought that when your teeth start to go, everything's going to go." (Non-Deprived)

CONCLUSIONS

The importance of these findings to decision making are wide ranging. One of the main features of using this kind of open-ended exploratory research procedure is that it gives the consumer a voice and does allow their priorities and perceived needs to be considered when setting the agenda. This study posed some interesting questions since it indicated that the type of dental services currently being encouraged by the dental profession are more consistent with the value systems of those from more affluent backgrounds than the values of those living in deprived communities. It therefore encourages dental practitioners to question their assumptions about what constitutes good dental practice. This re-assessment, or getting in touch with your consumer, is an essential process to go through for professionals working in the area of prevention where they are seeking to modify customer behaviour.

Another important benefit this type of analysis can bring to programme management and strategic thinking is a sense of realism; it enables planners to begin to set realistic and achievable targets. In this instance it was clear that the route of the problem (see figure 2) lay beyond the direct control of the health professional. The problem was not primarily service related but was rather culturally defined - it was due to differing social values and norms rather than to any specific short-comings with the services being offered.

Being able to set targets that are achievable is also important to morale since with preventive health programmes there are often over ambitious expectations of what can be achieved. This kind of research can help allay the anxieties of those charged with the responsibility for managing such programmes and puts into perspective the real advances that are being made.

As well as setting realistic targets this kind of applied research procedure can also be used to pin-point areas for action. With the dental study two areas were identified where improvements could be made to the existing services being offered. First, there was a problem with the professions image with customers having lost confidence in the dentists motives for offering treatment. Developing a system whereby payment and treatment are separated as currently happens with General Practitioners through the medical prescription system, may be one way of helping to restore confidence. Second, there was scope for improving the perceived service environment with many respondents claiming that the attitude of the dentist and the atmosphere in the dental surgery were responsible for arousing fear and anxiety.

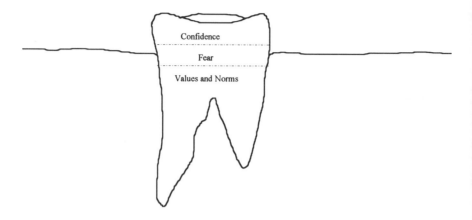

Figure 2. The root of the problem

Importantly, these problems have been recognised for some time and many changes have been made as a result. What appears to be happening in this instance, however, is that due to infrequent attendance users have only limited experience of modern dental services. Hence the fears that they express are to a larger degree based upon their experiences of the dentist as a child or when they were younger. This problem is further compounded by the fact that when such individuals do attend for treatment it is normally in a crisis situation where they are experiencing considerable pain and where the treatment given is often major and prolonged. This therefore only serves to reinforce their negative attitudes towards the service. In addition to this, there was also evidence to suggest that these patterns of behaviour and the fears and anxieties aroused by them could be being transmitted to their children and other family members.

The study results suggested that to break this cycle of fear (see figure 3) there is a need to continue to give school based dental education top priority and communications with the adult population should place less emphasis upon promoting dental check-ups as a means too better dental health and more upon them as a means of obtaining pain free dentistry.

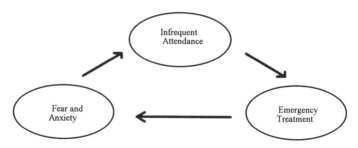

Figure 3. The Cylce of Fear

REFERENCES

Pitts, N.B. and Davies, J.A., 'Summary Report of 1987/8 Examination of 5-year-old children, *Scottish Health Boards Epidemilogical Programme.*

Royal Commission on the National Health Service Report, HMSO, London, 1979.

Scottish Health Priorities for the Eighties, Scottish Home and Health Department, HMSO, Edinburgh, 1986.

Todd, J.E., Walker, A.M. and Dodd, P. (1982), *Adult Dental Health, Vol 2, United Kingdom,* HMSO, London.

Todd, J.E. and Dodd, T. (1985), *Childrens dental health in the United Kingdom,* 1983, OPCS Social Surveys Division, HMSO, London.

Wallstron, B.S., Wallstron, K.A. (1978), *'Locus of control and health: a review of the literature,'* Health Education Monogr, 6, 107-117.

Weiss, J., Diserens, D. (1980), *'Health behaviour of dental professionals,'* Clin Prevention Dent, 2, 5-10.

Williams, A.F. (1972), *'Personality characteristics associated with preventive health practices,'* J Am Coll Dent, 39, 225-228.

10 Social Deprivation, Health Status and their Relationship on a Ward Basis in Camden and Islington

SANDRA SUBNER[1] & NIGEL BRUCE[2]

[1]Camden and Islington Health Authority
[2]University of Liverpool

INTRODUCTION

The recent NHS reforms have placed greater responsibility on district health authorities to identify the health care needs of its resident population in order to purchase appropriate health care services and allocate those purchases equitably. To perform these activities, information is required on the health status of the population and on existing inequalities in health service provision.

The aim of this study was to examine a link between deprivation and health status and to explore the usefulness of this type of analysis. The objectives were:

- To examine the relationship between three deprivation indices for the wards of Camden and Islington — Jarman, Townsend and Department of Environment (DOE).
- To assess the relationship between social deprivation as measured by the Jarman, Townsend and DOE indices, and mortality, morbidity and hospital utilisation rates on a ward basis in Camden and Islington.
- To assess the usefulness of deprivation indices in explaining variations in health status.

BACKGROUND

The Government's green paper the 'Health of the Nation' (1991) recognises that

> 'there are unacceptable variations in health status within society influenced by where we live, what social class we belong to, what job we do and which ethnic group we belong to' (DoH, 1991: 5).

Deprivation may be defined as:

Managerial Issues in the Reformed NHS. Edited by M.Malek, P.Vacani, J.Rasquinha & P.Davey
© 1993 John Wiley & Sons Ltd

'a state of .....disadvantage relative to the local community or the wider society or nation to which an individual, family or group belongs. People can be seen to be deprived if they lack the material standards of diet, clothing, housing, household facilities, working, environmental and locational conditions and facilities which are ordinarily available to their society and do not participate in or have access to the forms of employment, occupation, education, recreation, family and social activities and relationships which are commonly experienced or accepted'
(Benzeval *et al*, 1992).

Deprivation measures can contribute to the assessment of health need because there is a well established association between material deprivation and ill health (Black, 1980; Whitehead, 1987; Towsend *et al*, 1988). Deprivation measures can be used to identify communities where health care need is greater: communities where material resources are less and the capacity to cope with consequences of illness is less, and communities in which ill health is likely to be great in the future (Campbell *et al*, 1991).

DEFINING NEED

Two common definitions are given to the term 'health need' — 'the known ability to benefit from health care' (Stevens, Gabbay, 1991) and that which a person requires to stay in good health, which may include employment, nutrition, housing and access to social and health care services (Coventry, 1990). Health care needs can be defined as services that ought to be provided to improve the health of an individual or of a population. Irving (1983) believes that measuring the need for health services is made difficult by:

- Lack of medical consensus about an appropriate package of care for any specific condition,
- Difficulty of measuring the ability to benefit from an appropriate package of care,
- Definition of need varies over time and with the perceptions of individual clinicians,
- The scope for substituting different kinds of service.

A review of the literature suggests that there is still considerable debate concerning the measurement of deprivation. Measuring deprivation or underprivilege and determining its influence on health is complex and no single socio-economic variable or multiple index can sufficiently identify a 'special needs' area.

MEASURING DEPRIVATION

Current debate centres on the efficacy of the Jarman Underprivileged Area 8 score (UPA (8)) to measure deprivation. The Jarman index, constructed from the responses of general practitioners to a questionnaire asking how much they thought each of the 13 listed factors increased their workload, has been used as (i) a marker of deprivation in the consideration of social inequalities in health, (ii) as a tool by the Resource Allocation Working Party (RAWP) to review resource allocation and (iii) is currently being used to deliver special payments to general practitioners working in areas with underprivilege area scores over a certain value. In a recent article, Campbell *et al* (1991) criticized the UPA score as being inappropriate for use in allocating resources by health authorities for two reasons - one, that the Jarman index was not originally designed to be used as a measure of deprivation and two, the attempt to normalize the distribution of component variables has not worked well, with some variables such as ethnicity remaining skewed.

Other indices devised in an attempt to explain variation in health in terms of material deprivation include the Townsend Index, devised by Townsend *et al* (1988) in an analysis for the Northern region, and the Scottish Deprivation Development Index (SCOTDEP), developed by Morris and Carstairs (1991) for analysis of Scottish health data (Table 1).

Townsend's index comprises variables reflecting the absence of material

Table 1. Range of Variables for Indices of Deprivation

Variables	SCOTDP	JAR	TOWN	DOE	SDD
Unemployment	•	•	•	•	•
Youth Unemployment					•
No Car	•		•		
Low social class	•				
Unskilled		•			•
Overcrowding	•	•	•	•	
Below occupancy norm					•
Not owner occupied			•		
Lacking amenities				•	•
Single parent		•		•	•
Under age 5		•			
Elderly households					•
Lone pensioners		•		•	
1-year immigrants		•			
Ethnic Minorities		•		•	
Vacant dwellings				•	
Level and access (old)				•	
Level and access (<5)				•	
Permanent sickness				•	
Large households				•	

resources. Other commonly used measures are the Department of Environment (DOE) (six variable composite index which closely resembles Jarman's index) and the Scottish Development Department (SDD) (similar to Townsend's but substitutes social class for housing tenure) which were developed in relation to urban policy and planning. All of the indices are calculated using small area statistics from the 1981 Census.

Two recent studies have sought to compare the performance of the indices in relation to selected health indicators. A study undertaken by Campbell *et al* (1991) compared the Jarman (UPA (8)), the SDD and DOE indices and unemployment rates in respect of their correlation with measures of mortality and morbidity by electoral ward in a district. The measures used were the standardised mortality ratios (SMRs), admission rates (standardised and non-standardised) and permanent sickness rates. The authors found that the Jarman index had a lower correlation with measures of morbidity than did the other deprivation measures. In this study the correlation between unemployment as recorded in the 1981 Census and the deprivation indices was high. The authors have suggested that the unemployment rate in the community acts as a marker for both material and social deprivation and functions as a good proxy measure for deprivation.

The study carried out by Morris and Carstairs (1991) examined different indices in relation to their performance in explaining the variation observed in a range of health measures (see Figure 1), using data for postcode sectors in a range of health measures in Scotland. They concluded that both the Townsend and Scottish Deprivation Development indices performed well as measures of material deprivation in explaining variations in the health measures. The Jarman index was found to be less effective as a result of the inclusion of individual variables (under age 5, lone pensioners and ethnic minorities) which are seen to correlate very weakly, even negatively, with health indicators.

Standardised Mortality Ratios (SMRs)

Permanently sick

Temporarily sick

Standardized bed-days ratios

Standardized discharge ratios

Standardized mean stay

Figure 1. Measurement of Health Status

By what criteria should a deprivation index be selected? Campbell *et al* (1991) suggest that deprivation indices should be judged on their capacity to predict communities requiring health service provision. A deprivation index should be able to accurately identify an underprivileged area. In the attempt to assess the level of underprivilege among its residents, a health authority should select variables or a combination of variables which is most appropriate to the characteristics of that population. Although strong associations have been found to exist between deprivation and measures of mortality and morbidity, it is far too simplistic to state that the mere identification of underprivilege suggests the need for more health service provision.

MEASURING HEALTH STATUS

Health care needs are often determined on the basis of the health status of a particular group of individuals or of an entire population. Measures of health status can be divided into two categories - direct and indirect. Direct measures of health status can be 'disease-specific' in that they are based on the presence or absence of symptoms, physical signs and diagnosed disorders. Other direct measures could include 'self-reports' about health.

In trying to assess a link between deprivation and health care need, proxy measures of health status are often used. The proxy measure most commonly used is the SMR. The use of SMRs by the Resource Allocation Working Party heightened the debate about the use of mortality rates as proxy measures for morbidity and how accurately mortality indicates the relative needs for health care in a population. The RAWP formula used SMRs as a proxy measure for morbidity to take account of differences in the relative needs of the population for hospital care in excess of those explained by age and sex structures of the population. Mays (1986) has argued that the relatively high levels of morbidity which are experienced by 'deprived' populations may not be adequately reflected in the SMRs. Another criticism of the use of SMRs as a needs indicator is its insensitivity to the cause of a particular level of SMR i.e. a low SMR may reflect a low level of need (morbidity) or a high level of service effectiveness.

The paucity of data on health by ward makes selection of proxy measures of health difficult. For example, although it is possible to obtain standardised mortality ratios, either for those under 64 (premature mortality) or for all ages, it is difficult to obtain cause specific rates by electoral ward. This lack of information makes it difficult to ascertain the extent to which certain conditions contribute to a high or low SMR in a district and ward.

Data for this study are based on the resident population of the Hampstead and Bloomsbury and Islington Health Authorities, in the 46 electoral wards of the London boroughs of Camden and Islington. The area is also divided into 13 localities or neighbourhoods by the family health services authority.

The Camden and Islington populations are socially and economically heterogeneous. Islington has a relatively young population with the highest percentage of children in the two areas under the age of 15. South Camden has an older population with a greater proportion of persons over 65 years of age. A diverse minority ethnic community including Bengalis, Turks, Greeks, Africans, Chinese, Cypriots and Afro-Caribbeans is found in both areas. The minority ethnic community tends to be young with more than a fifth of its population under 15. Both districts are also increasingly becoming the place of residence for refugees from Somalia, Eritrea, Iraq, Turkey and Kurdistan. It is estimated that the Bloomsbury and Islington Health Authority has the greatest number of refugees, at 20 000 in the area covered by the North East Thames Regional Health Authority (NETRHA) (Karmi, 1992). A further 2,000 refugees are estimated to live in the area covered by the Hampstead Health Authority.

Affluence exists alongside deprivation within the districts (Appendices 1a — 1c). The mean Jarman score for the two health districts is 29.6 with a range from -0.97 to 46.78. Over two-thirds of the wards are above the national average. The most deprived ward is King's Cross (South Camden) and the least, Frognal in Hampstead. Five out of the ten most deprived wards fall within Islington while nine out of the ten most affluent wards are found in Hampstead.

METHODS

The link between deprivation and health status was examined on a ward basis. Although it would have been useful to examine the link between deprivation and health status at locality level rather than ward, the lack of postcoded data to allow enumeration district codes to be assigned makes this task difficult.

The first analysis undertaken was to test the hypothesis that there is a strong degree of association among the Jarman, Townsend and DOE indices. Pearson product-moment correlations were calculated using SPSS/PC+. The next series of analyses involved correlating the deprivation indices with the measures of health status. Standardised mortality ratios for all causes of death of Camden and Islington residents up to the age of 64 were calculated for each ward for the years 1985— 1989.

Five year rates for infant mortality, neonatal mortality and stillbirths were obtained for the years 1986—1990. Asthma and coronary heart disease were chosen to examine the usefulness of acute service utilisation. Asthma (children under age 5) and coronary heart disease (all ages) hospitalisation data representing finished episodes of treatment for the years 1990—1991 were obtained from the NETRHA's patient information system. Tuberculosis data were obtained from manual and computerised records of notifications for the period between September 1989 to December 1991. Notifications were postcoded and affixed an electoral ward code using a postcode grouper.

Pearson product-moment correlations with two-tailed significances were calculated for each deprivation index with each health measure. Scatterplots were drawn to illustrate any associations found between the deprivation indices and the various measures of health.

A mapping exercise was conducted to present the variation in health status across the two health districts.

RESULTS

The objectives of the analyses were to discover:

- the degree of interrelationship among the three deprivation indices; and

- what relationship (if any) exists among the deprivation indices and our seven criterion measures of health status.

The results are discussed in the following paragraphs.

A high degree of multicollinearity was found between the three deprivation indices (especially the Jarman and Townsend). Table 2 presents the results of the correlation analyses for the seven criterion measures of health status with the Jarman, Townsend and DOE index scores including 95% confidence intervals. Scatterplots for the Jarman analyses are shown in (Appendices 2a — 2g).

Table 2. Correlation between deprivation indices for 46 wards in Camden and Islington

	Deprivation Indices		
Indices	Jarman	Townsend	DOE
Jarman	*	0.911	0.823
Townsend	+0.911	*	0.874
DOE	+0.823	+0.874	*

+ (p = 0.00)

A preliminary investigation indicates that all three indices are positively correlated to a greater or lesser degree with the seven health status measures. As can be seen from Table 3, no single index was found to be significantly correlated to all seven health measures. In fact none of the deprivation variables were found to be significantly correlated with infant mortality rates or asthma for the 46 wards within Camden and Islington.

All three deprivation variables were significantly correlated with the standardised mortality ratios (all causes, under age 65) beyond the .01 level. Table 2 indicates us that any one of these variables alone would give the same information but the Townsend variable provides a slightly higher and more reliable estimate of the

Table 3. Correlation of deprivation indices with health measures
for the wards of Camden and Islington

	Measures of Health						
	SMR	Infant	Neonatal	Stillbirth	Asthma	Coronary	TB
Index							
JAR	0.558	0.196	0.288	0.356	0.180	0.255	0.414
	(.32 -.73)	(-.10 - .46)	(.00 - .53)	(.07 - .59)	(.12 - .45)	(-.04 - .51)	(.14 - .63)
	(p<0.00)	(p=0.19)	(p=0.05)	(p=0.02)	(p=0.23)	(p=0.09)	(p=0.00)
TOWN	0.609	0.131	0.188	0.275	0.174	0.354	0.385
	(.39 - .76)	(.17 - .41)	(.11 - .45)	(-.02 - .52)	(-.12 - .44)	(.07 - .58)	(.11 - .61)
	(p<0.00)	(p=0.38)	(p=0.21)	(p=0.07)	(p=0.25)	(p=0.02)	(p=0.01)
DOE	0.524	0.248	0.322	0.202	0.160	0.288	0.229
	(.28 - .71)	-.05 - .50)	(.04 - .56)	(.09 - .47)	(.14 - .43)	(-.00 - .53)	(-.07 - .49)
	(p<0.00)	(p=0.10)	(p=0.03)	(p=0.18)	(p=0.29)	(p=0.05)	(p=0.13)

Figures in parentheses are 95% confidence intervals.

relationship between deprivation and SMRs.

Four wards, King's Cross, Tollington, Highgate and Frognal were remarkable with respect to their deprivation score and the measures of health status. A short description of the wards highlighting particular features are given below.

King's Cross

A high level of social deprivation was found in this ward. It ranked first using the Jarman score, fourth with the Townsend index and seventeenth using the DOE index. A considerable, black and minority ethnic community constituting between 10 to 15% of the total population is found in the area. (1981 Census) The highest SMR (171) across the two districts was found in this ward. Low infant and neonatal mortality rates and stillbirths were recorded for this ward, 5.81/1 000, 4.36/1 000 and 1.45/1 000 respectively. 95% confidence intervals — infant (1.65 — 14.81), neonatal (0.92 — 12.6), stillbirths (0.06 — 8.12). King's Cross had the highest asthma hospital utilisation rate (25.46/1 000) for the two health districts - confidence interval (12.3 — 45.1). High TB notifications (1.56/1 000) were noted for this area - confidence interval (0.59 — 2.52).

Tollington

This ward also scored high on all three deprivation indices ranking second on the Jarman, fifth on the Townsend and fourth with the DOE. A large black and minority ethnic community (25 — 30%) is located in the area of the total population. A high SMR (151.7) and a high stillbirth rate (10.86/1 000) were noted. Infant and neonatal rates are average, 7.68/1 000 and 5.49/1 000 respectively. Confidence intervals were for infant (3.11 — 15.8) and neonatal (1.77 — 12.8).

Highgate

A relatively low deprivation score was found for this ward. It ranked near the bottom with the three indices. The black and minority ethnic population is less than 10%. High infant and neonatal mortality rates (20.22/1 000 and 12.44/1 000 respectively) were found for this ward. A high hospitalisation rate for asthma was noted - confidence interval (7.63 — 31.4).

Frognal

This Camden ward was found to be the least deprived ward in the two health districts. Low rates were found for all seven health measures.

Variations in health status across the two health districts are illustrated in Appendices 3 — 9.

DISCUSSION AND CONCLUSION

Our results suggest that any of the three indices — Jarman, Townsend and DOE could be used as a predictor variable when studying health status. The high degree of intercorrelation (especially between the Jarman and Townsend indices) had been noted by Morris and Carstairs in their 1991 comparative analysis (Table 4). Our findings also supported the contention made by Jarman, Townsend and Carstairs, 1991 that the indices intercorrelate strongly.

Table 4. Correlations between deprivation indices for Postcode Sectors in Scotland (Carstairs and Morris)

Indices	SCOTDEP	JAR	TOWN	DOEB	DOES	SSDEP
SCOTDEP	*					
JAR	0.826	*				
TOWN	0.960	0.801	*			
*DOEB	0.910	0.870	0.896	*		
*DOES	0.886	0.872	0.868	0.990	*	
*SDDEP	0.955	0.804	0.908	0.862	0.834	*

* SCOTDEP Developed by Carstairs and Morris for analysis of Scottish health data.
* DOEB Department of Environment measure developed mainly in relation to urban policies (Basic Index - unemployment has a weight of two)
* DOES Department of Environment measure developed mainly in relation to urban policies (Social Index - unemployment, single parents and lone pensioners have a weight of two)
* SDDEP Scottish Development Department measure developed mainly in relation to urban policies

The demographic and health data obtained and the maps produced illustrate the variation in social deprivation and health status across the two districts. Interpretation of the results must not be made without taking into account that the ward based data contains very small numbers which increases the effect of random variation.

The monitoring of morbidity and mortality on a small area basis should be a continuous process. Mortality data informs us of health outcomes reflecting in part the quality and level of care. Measuring deprivation in a district can highlight an area where perhaps closer examination and study is required. For example, in a ward with high morbidity and mortality rates, an investigation of the level and use of services by the residents could be undertaken. Relevant questions to be asked would include — do people make poor use of services, are services meeting demand, and are services appropriate, acceptable and accessible to all the residents of the area. Only after such research could it be determined whether extra resources are needed, or whether better use can be made of existing resources in order to improve health status.

This study did observe a relationship between social deprivation and premature mortality (all causes) as previously reported in national studies. In general, high deprivation scores were associated with high mortality and morbidity rates. No relationship was found to exist with measures of perinatal health - stillbirths and neonatal and infant mortality which is in contrast to other studies both nationally and internationally finding an association between low socio-economic status and high infant mortality rates (Baird and Thomson, 1969; Antonovsky and Berstein, 1977; Black, 1980; Blaxter, 1981). Surprisingly however, high neonatal and infant mortality rates were observed for the Highgate ward in Camden despite its relatively low deprivation score. In contrast, King's Cross had very low stillbirths, neonatal and infant mortality rates, despite being the most deprived ward in the districts. The findings do suggest the need for further study in the area of perinatal health including an examination of maternity and paediatric services - both community-based and hospital.

A relationship between hospital utilisation rates for asthma and coronary heart disease and social deprivation was not evident. This could be partly explained by the fact that hospital admission rates are influenced by general practitioners. High tuberculosis notification rates were found in three of the most deprived wards — Regent's Park, Somers Town and King's Cross — highlighting the need for targeted action to stem the rising number of cases in these areas. This preliminary investigation emphasises the need to obtain more information about pathways between mortality and morbidity in the community and the use of hospital services.

The usefulness of monitoring deprivation for the purposes of determining social and environmental conditions on health is mixed. Although it is important to measure the level of deprivation in an area, this factor alone cannot estimate or predict the need for health care. At this time, it is not possible to determine the contribution of social deprivation to the need for health care over and above that accounted for by morbidity. Even if such information were known, possible remedies to reduce deprivation among wards — both social and economic reform — which in turn might contribute to an improvement in health status, do not lie within the scope of the health service. Public health practitioners are left with the task of raising awareness among those individuals responsible for making reforms and ensuring that social deprivation and its link to health becomes part of the public agenda. Key individuals would include those who sit on joint planning committees between health and local authorities and those responsible for commissioning health care services for the local population.

This study has examined the relationship between social deprivation and seven measures of health status on a ward basis in two inner-city London boroughs that comprise the Hampstead and Bloomsbury and Islington health districts. Considerable variation in health status was found across the districts.

With the publication of the 'Health of the Nation', monitoring the health status of the population will be important to assess whether objectives in the five key areas are being met. It must be recognised that setting realistic and achievable targets to bring about changes in health status are difficult to formulate, partly because all determinants of health cannot be met or provided through the national health service, despite the demand to do so. In a speech last year, the former Chief Medical Officer of Health, Sir Donald Acheson, acknowledged that while health promotion initiatives seek to reduce risk factors such as smoking, poor diet and lack of physical activity, 'there is a limit to the extent to which improvements are likely to occur in the absence of a wider strategy to change the circumstances in which these risks arise by reducing deprivation and improving physical environment'. The work presented here may, with further development and refinement, provide a method of monitoring the vital task of reducing inequalities in health in a local population.

ACKNOWLEDGEMENTS

The assistance of the following individuals in- the preparation of this paper is gratefully acknowledged: Dr Ian Basnett, Dr Mark McCarthy, Alan Fleming, Dr Brenda Chipperfield, Jamil Choglay, Gerard Simms, Dan Altman and Rosalind Hann.

REFERENCES

Antonowsky, A. and Berstein, J. (1977), 'Social Class and Infant Mortality', *Soc Sci and Med.*, 11, 453.

Baird, D. and Thomson, A.M. (1969), 'General Factors Underlying Perinatal Mortality Rates', in Butler, R. and Alberman, E. D., *Perinatal Problems*, Livingstone, Edinburgh.

Benzeval, M., Judge, K. and Solomon, M. (1992), *The Health Status of Londoners: A Comparative Perspective*, King's Fund Institute, London.

Black, D. (1980), *Inequalities in Health: Report of a Working Group*, HMSO, London.

Blaxter, M. (1981), *'The Health of the Children: A Review of Research on the Place of Health in Cycles of Disadvantage*, Heinemann, London.

Campbell, D., Radford, J. and Burton, P. (1991), 'Unemployment Rates: An Alternative to the Jarman Index?' *British Medical Journal*, 303, 750-755.

Coventry Department of Public Health. (1990), *'Health in Coventry: Annual Report of the Coventry Health Authority'*, Coventry Health Authority, Coventry.

Department of Health. (1991), *'Health of the Nation: A Consultative Document for Health in England'*, HMSO, London.

Irving, D. (1983), *Identification of Underprivileged Areas (Technical Paper)*. London School of Economics, London.

Jarman, B., Townsend, P. and Carstairs, V. (1991), 'Deprivation Indices'. *British Medical Journal*, 303, 523.

Karmi, G. (1992), *Refugees in North West Thames and North East Thames Regional Health Authorities*, North West Thames Regional Health Authority, London.

Mays, N. (1986), *SMRs, Social Deprivation or What? Accounting for Morbidity in RAWP*. United Medical School of Guy's and St Thomas's Hospitals, London.

Morris, R. and Carstairs, V. (1991), 'Which Deprivation? A Comparison of Selected Deprivation Indexes,' *Journal of Public Health*, 13(4), 318-326.

Stevens, A. and Gabbay, J. (1991), 'Need Assessment Needs Assessment', *Health Trends*, 23, 20-23.

Townsend, P., Phillmore, P. and Beattie, A. (1988), *Health and Deprivation: Inequality and the North*, Croom Helm, London.

Whitehead, M. (1987), *The Health Divide: Inequalities in Health in the 1980's*, Health Education Authority, London.

Appendix 1a. Jarman U.P.A. Deprivation — Camden & Islington

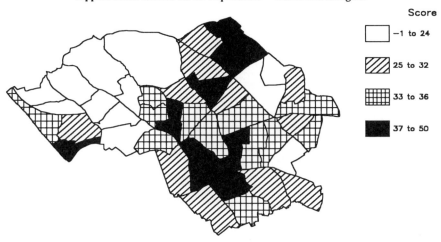

Score

-1 to 24

25 to 32

33 to 36

37 to 50

Appendix 1b. DOE Deprivation — Camden & Islington

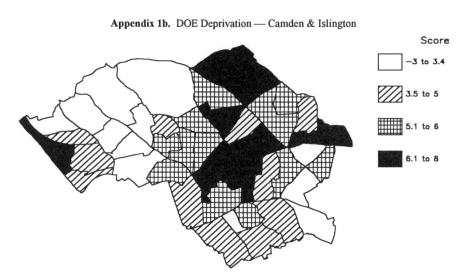

Score

-3 to 3.4

3.5 to 5

5.1 to 6

6.1 to 8

Appendix 1c. Townsend Material Deprivation — **Camden & Islington**

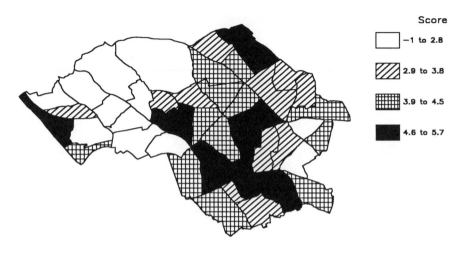

Appendix 2a. Jarman and SMR (1986—1989, ages 0—64)

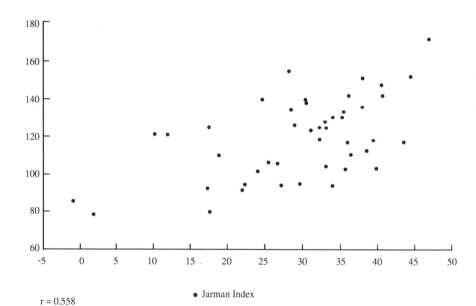

r = 0.558
(p = 0.00)

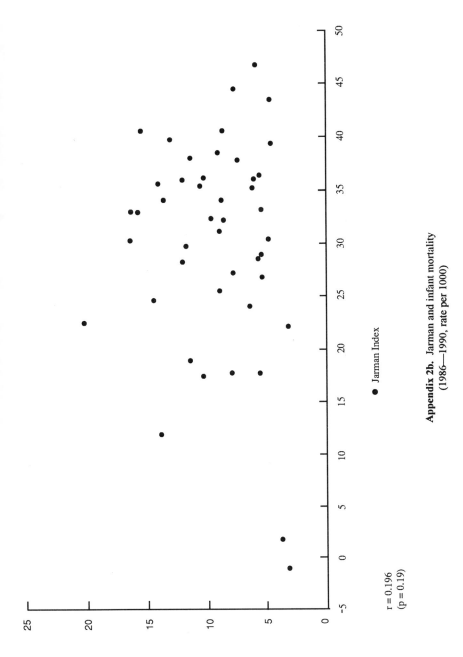

Appendix 2b. Jarman and infant mortality
(1986—1990, rate per 1000)

r = 0.196
(p = 0.19)

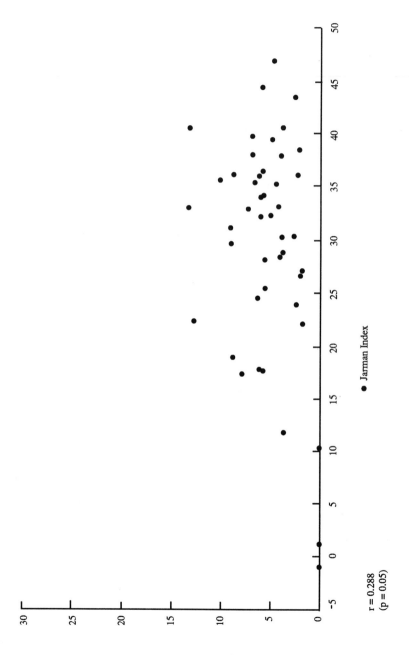

r = 0.288
(p = 0.05)

• Jarman Index

Appendix 2c. Jarman and neonatal mortality
(1986—1990, rate per 1000)

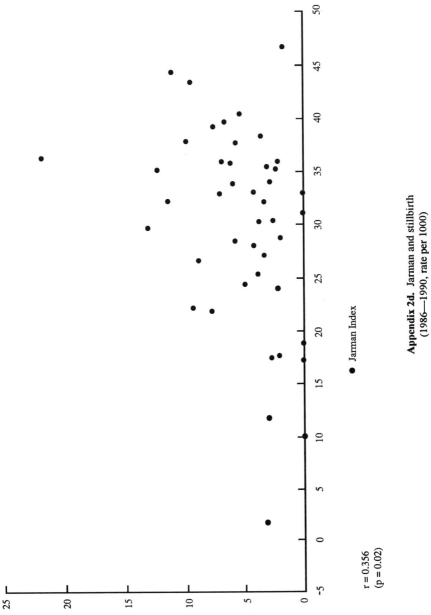

• Jarman Index

Appendix 2d. Jarman and stillbirth
(1986—1990, rate per 1000)

r = 0.356
(p = 0.02)

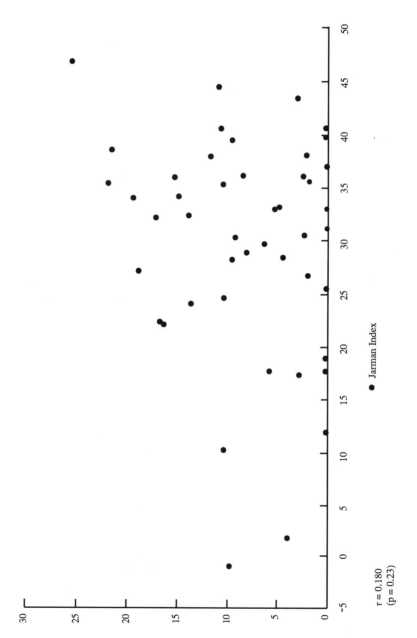

r = 0.180
(p = 0.23)

● Jarman Index

Appendix 2e. Jarman and asthma hospitalisation episodes
(1986—1990, rate per 1000)

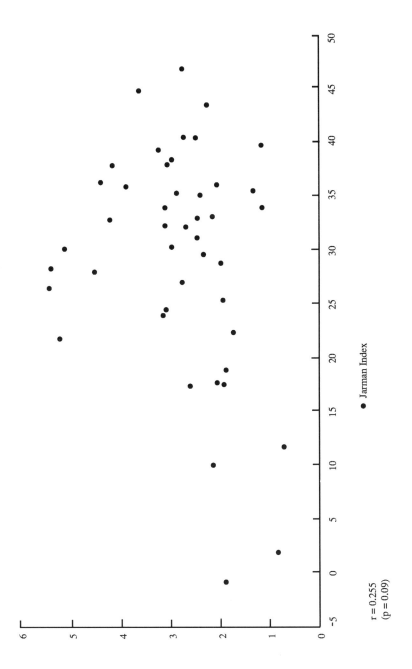

Appendix 2f. Jarman and coronary hospitalisation episodes
(finished episodes of treatment 1990/91)

● Jarman Index

r = 0.255
(p = 0.09)

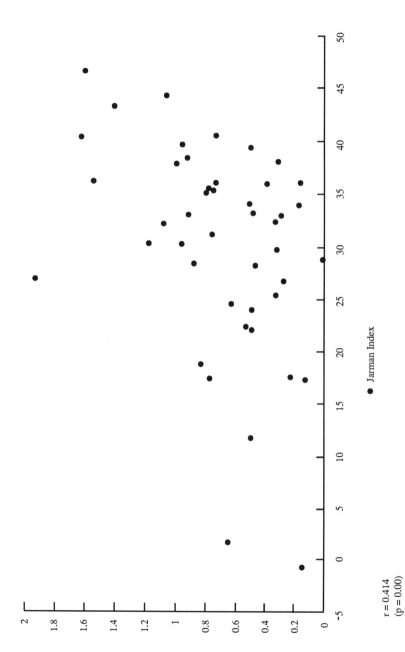

Appendix 2g. Jarman and tuberculosis notifications
(Sept 1989 — December 1991, rate per 1000)

● Jarman Index

r = 0.414
(p = 0.00)

Appendix 3. Standardised Mortality Ratio — All causes
(1985 — 1989, age 0 — 64)

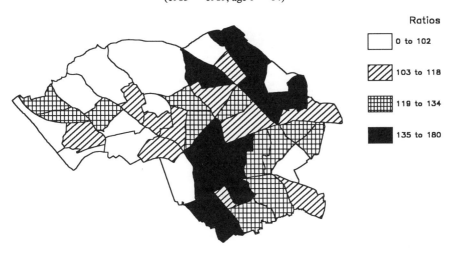

Ratios

☐ 0 to 102

▨ 103 to 118

▦ 119 to 134

■ 135 to 180

Appendix 4. Infant mortality (1986 — 1990)

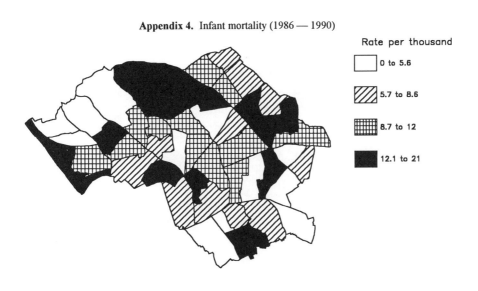

Rate per thousand

☐ 0 to 5.6

▨ 5.7 to 8.6

▦ 8.7 to 12

■ 12.1 to 21

Appendix 5. Neonatal mortality (1986 — 1990)

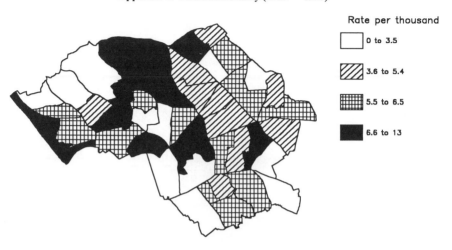

Rate per thousand

☐ 0 to 3.5

▨ 3.6 to 5.4

▦ 5.5 to 6.5

■ 6.6 to 13

Appendix 6. Stillbirth (1986 —1990)

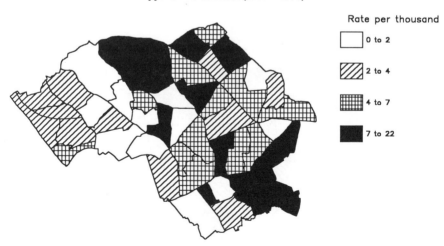

Rate per thousand

☐ 0 to 2

▨ 2 to 4

▦ 4 to 7

■ 7 to 22

Appendix 7. Asthma hospitalisation episodes
(1990/91, age 0 — 4)

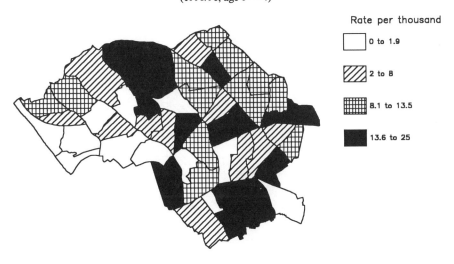

Rate per thousand

☐ 0 to 1.9

▧ 2 to 8

▦ 8.1 to 13.5

■ 13.6 to 25

Appendix 8. CHD hospitalisation episodes
(all ages 1990/91)

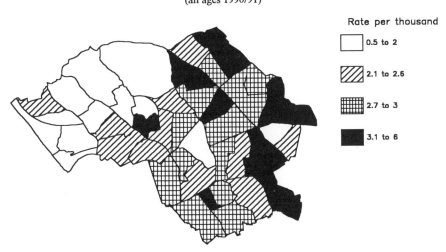

Rate per thousand

☐ 0.5 to 2

▧ 2.1 to 2.6

▦ 2.7 to 3

■ 3.1 to 6

Managerial Issues in the Reformed NHS

Appendix 9. Tuberculosis notifications
Camden & Islington, September 1989 — December 1991

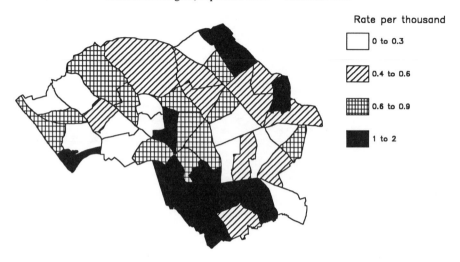

11 Patient Defined Audit — A New Perspective

LOUISE BELL[1], REVA BERMAN BROWN[2] & SEAN MCCARTNEY[2]

1 Southend Community Care Services NHS Trust
2 University of Essex

INTRODUCTION

The paper argues that audit in the healthcare field is likely to prove more effective if the views of the service users (those people who are consumers of healthcare services) are taken into consideration when devising audit tools. Articles that refer to auditing in the healthcare field (Berwick, 1989; Bunker, 1990, Chassin et al, 1986) look at medical audit and advise as to suitable methods to implement it. But other fields in healthcare are also beginning to implement audit processes as a way of looking at the care that they are providing. There is still, however, little work on user-definition of the elements that are contained within a healthcare audit tool, based on customers' perceptions of a quality service. The paper provides the preliminary results of an empirical investigation into the perceptions of service users. The ultimate aim of the research is to incorporate effective definitions of patient-defined quality within a healthcare audit tool.

THE CONTEXT OF AUDIT IN HEALTH CARE

The subject and practice of audit is one of the many issues being pursued in the current agenda for change in the National Health Service (NHS). Audit, in the sense of the general assessment and evaluation of healthcare, has always been practised to some extent in the healthcare field. The idea of carrying out some activity and then evaluating its impact is not new. What is a departure is current practice, as represented in the definition of medical audit in the NHS Review White Paper (1989) which requires the systematic, critical analysis of the quality of medical care, including the procedures used for diagnosis and treatment, the use of resources, and the resulting outcome and quality of life for the patient.

Managerial Issues in the Reformed NHS. Edited by M.Malek, P.Vacani, J.Rasquinha & P.Davey
© 1993 John Wiley & Sons Ltd

Medical audit (referring to the audit of care provided by doctors) has now become an expected part of routine professional practice for all clinician working in the NHS, and an organizational structure and sets of procedures have been developed, aided by financial support from the Department of Health (Moss, 1992).

A parallel development has been seen in clinical audit, which is becoming an expected process amongst other professional groups (Goldstone and Doggett, 1989).There have been a number of Government initiatives for healthcare quality improvement, and audit is seen as one tool which can be utilised to ensure that patients receive a care package which helps to improve the mix of effectiveness, efficiency, adequacy, and scientific-technical quality (Vouri, 1982).

Audit has come to the fore in the UK healthcare field as a means of monitoring the care provided, and establishing new standards for practice. In the main, however, the development has focused on two distinct areas: managerial and professional audit. Managerial audit can be seen to be largely concerned with the use of resources in the provision of healthcare in the NHS, and appears to have been largely stimulated by resource management and value for money ideas. Professional audit is concerned with areas which appertain to standards that are acceptable for professional practice, for example relating to acceptable standards required for the prescription of medications (Doyal, 1992). Managerial perspectives do not adequately consider the quality of care because they do not actively involve the professionals who provide it. The professional approach is limited because it focuses on each profession independently and is based on peer review, not customer views.

Little progress has been made towards the active inclusion of the patients' views, yet current Government views as expressed through various customer charters and increasing consumerism pressures all indicate the need to make the patient central to thinking about quality. While satisfaction surveys are fairly common, in general they reflect the designer's view of what is important, and although they indicate levels of satisfaction with a whole variety of issues, they provide little indication of whether or not these issues are important (Morris, 1990. What is needed, as well as the managerial or professional view of what is appropriate is an audit tool which reflects what patients require or expect. The development of such a tool is being undertaken in Southend Community Care Services NHS Trust as a two-year project sponsored by the North East Thames Regional Health Authority.

RESEARCH DESIGN

The research is undertaken in two stages: the first stage, is to elicit from a sample of healthcare users, their perceptions of quality healthcare service. From these perceptions, an audit tool can be devised which, should enable the audit of the many different professions within the health service. The assumption underlying this intention is that quality, defined by the user, implicitly contains information that will remain constant whichever service the user will visit.

The research examines the issue of auditing from a new perspective that focuses solely on the views of the service user. This approach has been made viable by means of the use of two already-validated research instruments: the Parasuraman *et al* (1988) Servqual instrument, which measures customer expectation versus perception, prior and subsequent to an encounter with any service, and the Heywood-Farmer and Stuart (1987) instrument, which looks at professional service quality, and was originally used to audit the quality of service provided by GPs.

These research instruments were specially adapted for use in the health field by including data taken from critical focus group interviews, individual interviews and open-ended qualitative questions. The focus was the question: "What do you think quality from health services means ?" A questionnaire was devised and piloted on several occasions and subsequently adjusted.

It was felt unwise to assume that there are generally-held views across all types and ages of patients, and that therefore the initial research work should focus on a specific group of patients. Given the large and growing numbers of people aged over 75, and their comparative neglect in the literature (Block, 1974; Loudon, 1976; Petre, 1986), the sample chosen for the research was health services provided for the over-75s. The sample (n = 210) was taken from the general population, and were all aged over 75, on or after 1st November, 1991. All subjects are on the books of one of seven general practices in the Southend Community Care Services NHS Trust, and were selected by their general practitioners, using random selection tables to provide equal numbers of males and females. The rationale behind the choice of this age-group is that there is an increase in the ageing population in the UK, which has resulted in a marked increase in the total amount spent on healthcare for this age group. The development of an audit tool which would indicate whether or not such care is effective and of good quality, is likely to result in both savings in cost and improvements in service delivery.

The questionnaire was administered in two ways: by means of face-to-face interviews and through the mail. Of the 120 subjects selected to be interviewed, 90 responded, and 61 agreed to participate in the research, giving a response rate of 68%. Five of the interview subjects were reported by their families or their GPs to have died between the time of their selection and the sending out of the questionnaire, and 19 refused to participate. A total of 90 postal surveys were sent out. Of the 60 questionnaires mailed with an incentive to reply, 41 were returned, and of the 30 questionnaires posted with no incentive, 21 were returned, making a total of 62, giving a response rate of 69%. Thus, 123 out of the sample of 210 participated in the research, a response rate of 68%.

The high response rate may be put down to the possibility that this age group hold their local GP in high esteem and that they responded because they felt obliged to, or that they are interested in the subject because the healthcare they receive is important to them, or that they felt that they wanted to voice their opinions, seldom asked for from people of their age. The preliminary results from the responses appear to confirm the viability of the second stage of the research, which is to devise an audit tool that can be used in a variety of healthcare situations. Because the findings currently reached reveal that service users' expectations of a service differ from those discussed in the quality literature that takes managerial and professional perspectives as their focus (Berwick *et al*, 1992; McNicol, 1992; Maxwell, 1984), the paper next discusses a number of issues contained in the literature on marketing, services and audit in health.

MARKETING, SERVICES AND AUDIT

The current view of the healthcare system in the UK is that it needs to become more market-oriented in the climate of NHS Trusts and GP Fundholders, who will be buying and selling a variety of health services. This is a conscious attempt to create a more competitive and market driven health service.

The customer will, it is hoped, become more important in this process, which will become increasingly transaction-based, in a similar way to those transactions encountered in any other service industry, such as banks or solicitors. Marketing literature is highly developed and has a well-researched knowledge-base that has been established over many years. The need to succeed in the business arena has risen due to increased competition from numerous sources. Marketing literature has looked into the elements that consumers define as quality areas and has produced several solutions in response to this increase in competition. In particular, the marketing literature has needed to address the rise in service industries world-wide and the concurrent decline in manufacturing industries. It has defined the differences between the manufacturers and service providers and has explored the issues that differentiate between a successful and an unsuccessful company. The links between these issues/dilemmas in the marketing arena can be related to the NHS, which is a service industry that is having to become increasingly aware of market trends. It faces increased competition from the private sector, and other sectors that are providing more cost-effective services or better quality services.

The difference between a successful and an unsuccessful NHS trust may lie in the way in which one trust may be able to satisfy all its customers, gain contracts and increase revenue, and another may fail to do these things and, as a business concern, may be completely unsuccessful. This is likely to result in the cutting of services and the particular trust that is not competing in the market will fail. This has not occurred as yet, but the need to prevent this occurring will mean that the views, wishes and opinions of the customers must be valued and taken into consideration. Therefore, patient-defined audit tools must become a reality and can no longer be avoided by professionals and managers. There is increasing emphasis on the dictum that the customer is always right, and customers' views will be coming to the forefront with recent government initiatives such as the Patients' Charter.

The nature of service industries is that they have direct contact with consumers of the service. The proliferation of service industries in the developed world means that in order to succeed, companies need to provide a good quality service that customers will recommend and will use again. There is a large body of literature concerning services, and quality in services, topics researched include areas such as the problems of defining service quality (Edvardsson, 1988, Voss *et al*, 1985), the classification of services (Lovelock, 1983), the measurement of customers' perceptions of quality

(Parasuraman *et al*, 1988), and the essential nature of customer satisfaction in any provision of service quality (Gronroos, 1984, Johnston, 1987).

THE ROLE AND IMPLEMENTATION OF AUDIT IN HEALTHCARE

Many of the articles that refer to auditing in the healthcare field (Chassin *et al*, 1986; Bunker, 1990; Berwick, 1989) look at medical audit and advise as to suitable methods of implementation/improvement. Other groups in healthcare are also beginning to implement audit processes as a way of looking at the care/services they are providing and this is beginning to become a requirement in many services. Generally, audit is approached in a mechanistic way, following professional or fiscal guidelines. Auditing, however, is not an end in and of itself; it exists to improve the quality of care delivered and, as stated in the Patients' Charter, it is imperative that the views of the service users are taken into account.

The implementation of audit throughout the health service has been a process with regional variations which have created some centres of excellence but also some centres where there exists fairly low-key approach to audit. These variations are the result of the nature of quality as a specialism in health, which is still a new field of knowledge. Professional and managerial audit tools already exist, and these tend to dictate the route being taken in the definition of quality and of audit in the healthcare field. Existing professional standards of service are applied to areas such as the quality of treatment/care. Managerial audit tools tend to be used, approaching audit from a cost/benefit aspect or from looking for the successful achievement of specified service standards.

FINDINGS

The questionnaire began with the usual demographic questions relating to social class, family and marital status of the sample. These questions were included in order to be able to assess whether these factors had any bearing on what patients consider quality to be. The demographic information elicited is shown in Table 1.

The responses were subjected to a factor analysis which revealed that there were no underlying trends or factors contained within the data. Tests for correlation revealed that there were low correlations between the different variables. No strong associations or patterns were found. This suggests that the items on the questionnaire are independent, with no overlap or inter-relationship between the various categories. the responses indicate, however, that all the items are important to the respondents. All the variables were subjected to independent t-tests, which look at the effects of two groups on a single variable. The t-tests revealed that for all variables, gender had no effect on respondent replies. The t-test was also used to assess the effects of being married or being alone. This was also found to be of no significance.

Table 1. Demographic information

SOCIAL CLASS of respondents	
1	11.7%
2	8.1%
3	21.6%
4	24.3%
5	19.8%
Housewife	4.5%

FAMILY RELATIONSHIPS of respondents	
Have children only	7.2%
Have grandchildren only	8.1%
Have children, grandchildren and great-grandchildren	61.3%
Have none of the above	25.2%

MARITAL STATUS of respondents	
Single	2.7%
Married	44.1%
Widowed	51.4%
Divorced	1.8%

The LIVING ARRANGEMENTS of respondents	
Flat	22.5%
Bungalow	36.0%
Warden-run accommodation	5.4%
Residential accommodation	0.9%

The year of birth of respondents ranged from 1896 to 1918.
The gender of respondents: Male 49.5% and Female 50.5%

DETERMINING QUALITY

The Griffiths Report (1983) on the management structure within the NHS provided a stimulus to those who believe that patients' views of the health services they receive should be actively sought.   Among Griffiths' recommendations was that a more systematic method should be implemented in order to take account of patients' views. This is what this study is seeking to establish.

The preliminary findings of the analysis of the respondent sample's views have enabled the building up of a picture of the patients' perspectives of what quality in healthcare means to them. This picture highlights the inadequacies of the audit tools that exist at present and suggest that it is counter-productive to ignore such views when developing any audit tool with claims to effectiveness.

McNicol (1992) suggests seven components that comprise a quality service as:

1.   ACCEPTABILITY — The service offered must be acceptable to both patients and staff. The needs of patients are pre-eminent, but the service must also be acceptable to the staff who provide it.
2.   PROMPTNESS — The service should be available with the minimum of delay.

3. RELEVANCE — The service must meet the needs of patients rather than those of the professionals who provide it.
4. INFORMATION — Information about the treatment and the likely outcomes must be provided.
5. RESPECT FOR PATIENT CHOICE — The patient must be given adequate information so as to enable him/her to make informed choices.
6. TECHNICAL QUALITY — The highest possible degree of technical quality must be reached, and we must improve our methods of measurement so that we can be confident about the outcomes.
7. COST EFFECTIVENESS — The need to provide good value for money must be accepted.

Maxwell (1984) described six facets of quality service in healthcare and discussed these in a subsequent article (1992). These have been useful, in the health field, at several levels, both practically and conceptually. Maxwell's six facets give rise to questions about their implementation:

1. EFFECTIVENESS — Does the treatment give the best that is available in the technical sense, according to those best equipped to judge? What is their evidence? What was the overall result of the treatment?
2. ACCEPTABILITY — How humanely and considerately is the treatment/service delivered? What does the patient think of it? What is the setting like? Are privacy and confidentiality safeguarded?
3. EFFICIENCY — Is the output maximised for given input? How does the cost of the treatment compare with the cost of the same treatment by another, similar unit of delivery?
4. ACCESS — Can people get this treatment/service when they need it?
5. EQUITY — Is this patient or group of patients being fairly treated in comparison with others?
6. RELEVANCE — Is the overall pattern and balance of services the best that could be achieved, taking into account the needs and wants of the population as a whole?

In the main, despite certain differences in terminology, McNicol's list parallels Maxwell's — McNicol's Technical Competence is Maxwell's Effectiveness, and his Respect For Patient Choice is Maxwell's Effectiveness.

While the respondents' perceptions of quality echo many of these facets, their emphasis is different, and it is suggested, this difference should be taken into account when developing an audit tool for healthcare. For instance, while they echoed McNicol's Respect criterion in stating that they want "to be told the truth" about their condition, they gave more priority to criteria that neither Maxwell nor McNicol have mentioned, such as "feeling that staff believe what they say" and "feeling free to ask questions, without being regarded as a nuisance". Table 2 gives the frequencies of items which the respondents perceive as indicative of quality of healthcare service.

Table 2. Respondent Perceptions of Quality Service

It matters to me to —	
— be told the truth about my condition	95%
— feel that the staff are interested me	94%
— feel that the staff have my best interests at heart	94%
— know that tasks will be performed as promised (eg. phoning when stated)	94%
— feel that staff believe what I say	92%
— be treated with respect	91%
— wait in areas that are pleasant and comfortable	91%
— know that the equipment used is up-to-date	90%
— have easy-to-follow signs indicating where to go	90%
— be given help when I ask, and not be fobbed off	90%
— be notified of changes to my treatment	90%
— be seen and talked to in private	86%
— know when follow-up visits are arranged	85%
— feel free to ask questions without regarded as a nuisance	84%
— have access to lifts rather than stairs	82%
— have written information about my condition	75%
— be notified of the time I will be seen	70%
— be informed of what is going to happen to me	70%

The questionnaire was built around a 5-point scale ranging from "matters very much indeed" to "doesn't matter at all". The percentages below refer to a conflation of the two categories "matters very much indeed" and "matters greatly".

CONCLUSION

It is believed that an audit tool which has built into it the perceptions of the service user, such as those elicited in this research, will be assured of validity, and will not be measuring the wrong things in the wrong way.

The next stage of the study is to devise an audit tool which is a true measure against which to explore the service user's actual perceptions during contact with a specific provider of healthcare. These perceptions can then be measured against expectations and the two can be compared to elicit information about whether or not a service is meeting customer requirements.

REFERENCES

Berwick, D., (1989) 'Continuous improvements as an ideal in healthcare', New England Journal of Medicine, Vol. 320, pp. 53-56.

Block, J., (1974) 'The Aged consumer and the Marketplace: A Critical Review', Marquette Business Review, Vol. 18, No. 2, pp.73-81.

Bunker, E., (1990) 'Variations in hospital admissions and the appropriateness of care: American preoccupations', British Medical Journal, Vol. 301, pp. 531-532.

Chassin, M., Brook, R. H., Park, R. E., Keesey, J., Sink, A., Kosecoss, J., Kahn, K., Merick, N. and Soliman, D. H., (1986) 'Variations in the use of medical surgical services by the Medicare population', New England Journal of Medicine, Vol. 314, pp. 285-290.

Doyal, L., (1992) 'The need for moral audit in evaluating quality in healthcare', Quality in Healthcare, September, Vol. 1, pp.178-183.

Edvardsson, B., (1988) 'Service Quality in Customer Relationships', Service Industries Journal, Vol. 8, No. 4.

Goldstone, L. and Doggett, D., (1989) Monitor, Leeds: Poly Enterprises.

Gronroos, C.,(1984) 'A Service Quality Model and Its Marketing Implications', European Journal of Marketing, Vol. 18, No. 4.

Haywood-Farmer, J. and Stuart, I, (1992) Services Plus: Effective Service Management, Quebec: Morin Publisher Ltd.

Johnston, R., (1983) 'A framework for developing a quality strategy in a customer processing operation', University of Warwick Working Paper.

Lovelock, C., (1983) 'Classifying Services to Gain Strategic Marketing Insights', Journal of Marketing, Vol. 47, No. 1, pp. 9-20.

Loudon, L., (1976) 'The Senior Citizen: An Underdeveloped Market Segment', Southern Marketing Proceedings, pp.124-126.

McNicol, M., (1992) 'Achieving Quality Improvement by Structured Patient Management', Quality in Healthcare, Vol. 1, No. 3, (Supplement) pp. 40-41.

Maxwell, R. (1984) 'Quality Assessment in Health', British Medical Journal, Vol. 288, pp. 1470-1472.

Maxwell, R. (1992) 'Dimensions of Quality Revisited: From Thought to Action', Quality in Healthcare, Vol. 1, p. 173.

Morris, B., (1990) 'Incorporating Customer Requirements in Healthcare', Paper presented at the Conference on Total Quality Management in Healthcare, Birmingham, October.

Moss, F., (1992) 'Achieving Quality in Hospital Practice', Quality in Healthcare, Vol. 1, pp. 17-19.

Parasuraman, A., Zeithaml, V., and Berry, L., (1988) 'Servqual: A multiple-item scale for measuring consumer perception of service quality', Journal of Retailing, Spring, Vol. 64, No. 1, pp. 12-40.

Petre, P., (1986) 'Marketeers Mine for Gold in the Old', Fortune International, March, pp. 48-54.

Voss, C., (1985) Operations Management in Service Industries and the Public Sector, London: John Wiley and Sons.

Vouri, H., (1982) 'Scandinavian Model Healthcare Programmes - A Cousin of Quality Assurance', International Journal of Healthcare Quality Assurance, Vol. 2, No. 1.

12 Quality, Ideology and Consumer Choice — Health Care Standards and Stakeholder Participation

WENDY J. GREGORY & MICHAEL P. WALSH

University of Hull

INTRODUCTION

During the last decade or so Britain has been gripped by a growing demand for improved "quality" in products and services. The manufacturing and commercial sectors have recently been joined by public sector service organisations wishing to capitalise on quality schemes which purport to provide enormous gains for vendor and purchaser alike. Government reforms in the National Health Service (NHS), one such public sector organisation, have introduced a system of health provision which has arguably interposed a "purchaser" between the service provider and the user. This paper explores the development and use of quality ideas within the NHS in relation to these structural changes. A strategy is proposed for ensuring the continuation of the central quality philosophy of "meeting customer's requirements" within the NHS which allows the user of the service to be the defined customer together with the new, Government-created "purchasers".

Before we can begin to reflect upon the methods for ensuring the status of the NHS user as "Customer-King", it is necessary to discuss the introduction and utility of quality related concepts within the NHS. The traditional domain of quality ideas is that of industrial organisations, which we will now consider.

AN INDUSTRIAL VIEW OF "QUALITY"

Quality is used in a variety of differing contexts, and has a number of meanings arising from these. Some common definitions are associated with the group of experts on quality in industry, popularly known as "quality gurus". Three examples from Munro-Faure and Munro-Faure (1992) are Taguchi's "Quality is the loss imparted to society after the good is shipped", Juran's "Quality is fitness for use or purpose" and Crosby's "Quality is conformance to requirements".

Managerial Issues in the Reformed NHS. Edited by M.Malek, P.Vacani, J.Rasquinha & P.Davey
© 1993 John Wiley & Sons Ltd

Other quality definitions are given by the British Standards Institute (BSI). Their most recent definition, supported by Oakland (1989), states that quality is "simply meeting customer requirements". The point that Oakland makes is that quality is in the eye of the beholder, and that what some people would find an acceptable good or service, others would not. This means that "excellent" attributes of a product or service do not equate with its intrinsic quality unless previously specified as requirements by the customer.

Along with these difficulties in pinning down a clear definition of quality, writers have recently focused on identifying who is the customer of the system: i.e. who defines what is the quality of a product or service.

AN INDUSTRIAL VIEW OF THE "CUSTOMER"

The term "customer" has two interpretations: "internal" customers are employees or departments of a business or organisation who receive some output from other employees or departments; "external" customers are those people or organisations who buy the end product or service of the business. It can be seen that the customer forms one part of an interaction, in which the word quality has great significance.

We intend to focus on the latter use of the term in which the customer is extrinsic to the organisation providing the product or service. Our intention here is to highlight the fact that current restructuring of the British health care system gives rise to an increased diversity in the customers that the system serves. Hospitals will be competing for business from health authority funded "purchasers". Clearly, such large scale "customers" have far more clout than the individual, who will be further removed from the system of provision. An issue raised by this is how the user can maintain any impact on the methods for defining quality following the introduction of the new structure.

This is a point we will elaborate upon later. A different question raised by the recognition of the new competitive arena concerns the ideological bases of quality initiatives, to which we now turn.

INDUSTRIAL QUALITY IDEOLOGY

The Board of Trade (formerly the Department of Trade and Industry) maintains that, in meeting customer requirements, quality management provides the most important competitive edge for contemporary industrial enterprises (Department of Trade and Industry, 1991). Since success (and profitability) is taken as a categorical imperative, it follows that managers *should* use quality ideas to strive for "competitive advantage". Ideologically, then, quality initiatives in industry are linked to the capitalist framework for market operations. The ideological principle of quality in capitalism is therefore that "quality is good for your bottom line".

An alternative view raises the possibility of connecting quality imperatives to broader, societal needs. This view holds that "Quality is the loss imparted to society after the good is shipped" (Taguchi, 1979). If the loss is low, then quality is high and *vice versa*. Since Taguchi does not specify the types of losses that may detract from the quality of a product or service the door is opened for issues such as environmental degradation, equity, and the destruction of natural resources to be admitted into the discussion arena. There is clearly scope here for a radically different ideological base to that proposed in the capitalist market model.

This is not the only distinguishing feature of Taguchi's quality philosophy. By introducing a time dimension he highlights the point that the loss may not be experienced contemporaneously with the purchase of the good or service. Those who define quality must look out for the interests of others who would not normally be considered at all, future generations. Clearly, this view is more sophisticated than "simply meeting customer requirements".

Notwithstanding the foregoing, it is difficult to identify a purely altruistic quality ideology in the commercial literature, whilst it can be argued that altruism underlies many individuals' motives for working within the NHS. Adopting a quality ideology such as that of "meeting customer's requirements" would clearly generate tensions for people predisposed to a differing culture. Similarly, Taguchi's perspective could be at odds with a health care system that has not previously had to publicly account for the losses likely to be experienced by others through provision of any of its services.

These tensions bear some further consideration that may lead to the development of an alternative quality ideology that is more consistent with the founding principles of the NHS. Firstly, it is worthwhile exploring the context in which such tensions have arisen.

THE DEVELOPMENT OF "MARKETS" IN THE NHS

Since the inception of the NHS in 1948, its principle business has been health care for the nation, paid for by taxation and free at the point of delivery. There has been, however, a history of public anxiety about the NHS, and a perception that it was, and is, "inefficient". To some people it appears to waste resources, and there are frequent scandals. Despite this history it came as a surprise to her cabinet in January 1988 when, according to Maynard (1992), the Conservative Prime Minister, Margaret Thatcher, unilaterally announced a comprehensive reform of the NHS on national television.

The Conservative Government under Margaret Thatcher was noted for its strongly ideological position on the "freedom of markets". It is therefore hardly surprising that the type of reform implemented instituted the so-called "internal market" in which purchasing of NHS services was separated from the provision or use of services. This was done by facilitating and encouraging the change of service units into autonomous NHS Trusts. Additionally, purchasers of NHS services, including newly created fund-holding GPs, could negotiate contracts with any provider of a service, including non-NHS profit making providers. The NHS reform was therefore wholly congruent with the Government's drive for improved "value for money" from public services.

"Value for money" is a phrase that is frequently used by the Government about public services of all kinds. Since "added-value" and "quality" are used more or less interchangeably the motivation to adopt a "quality management" approach was significantly advanced. This was further compounded by the system of contracts between purchasers and providers which required quality specifications. A competitive motive was thus generated amongst providers since winning contracts meant winning revenue, and losing contracts meant losing revenue. The Government anticipated that competition for contracts amongst providers would drive up quality, drive down prices, and demonstrably improve "value for money".

The ideological and philosophical commitment to a quality oriented market place within the NHS was in place: what needed to follow were some pragmatic guidelines concerning implementation of the reforms.

QUALITY IN THE NHS

The implications of the 1989 reforms for quality in the NHS were indicated by the Government White Paper "Working For Patients" which boldly stated that "In short, every hospital in the NHS should offer what the best offer now" (HMSO, 1989, paragraph 1.14). This appeared to imply that there exists some objective specification to which NHS hospitals could aspire in offering "the best". What is not clear from the White Paper is by what criteria, and by whom, hospitals are to be judged.

A number of different sets of criteria have been suggested by various quality writers. The most well known views of quality in the NHS are those of Maxwell (1984) and Donabedian (1980) whose methods of quality assessment involve standard setting according to formulae. Here quality is defined and achieved when detailed quantitative and qualitative specifications are met. These two approaches to quality are used widely in the NHS, for example in "managing the nursing resource" (Rainbow, 1991). Furthermore, they accord with the imperative of quality specifications in contracts between purchasing authorities and independent units (HMSO, 1989).

With these developments, quality is now both formally and permanently on the agenda.

"QUALITY" AND "CUSTOMER" IN THE NHS

There is an ambiguity here in the use of the term "quality". It is being used to describe specifications in a contract for which a suitable price can be negotiated. It is also being used to describe the purchaser's satisfaction with the transaction. Whichever way quality is used in the internal "provider" market of the NHS, the customers are the purchasing authorities because they hold the funds, and it is their requirements that providers seek to satisfy. The user of the NHS has no direct control over specifications in contracts put out to tender, nor over purchasing decisions. The NHS user (the patient) is no longer the NHS customer. In the new model of health provision the customer and the user are separated.

The significance of the separation of the users and customers of the NHS is that quality can be perceived in many different ways. To provide an example of the kinds of positions that might be adopted, we can imagine *providers* to whom quality could mean "providing the best possible solution for each client, no matter what"; *purchasers* to whom it could mean "meeting specification" at the lowest possible price; and *users* to whom it could mean "having the largest amount of choice in health care options, regardless of cost". Clearly these perceptions may or may not match one another, and we have specifically chosen viewpoints that seem antithetical to illustrate the case. Many other variations will exist.

By introducing another actor into the health care system, the purchaser, the Government has sought to provide an "unbiased" evaluator of NHS services - a judge of quality. Quality is no longer a subjective experience of the end user, but some purportedly "objective" criterion of an uninvolved third party. There will be no tensions generated when purchaser definitions of quality match with those of the user, but sufficient evidence of the plurality of user views on health and illness exists to suggest that a precise match is unlikely. It is this plurality of perspectives that we are seeking to address in our current research, and which we return to later in the paper.

Of course, there is a danger here of talking about patient-users as though all patients form some homogenous mass capable of defining quality in relation to health care provision. There is, however, a great deal of evidence that patient-users are not homogenous, and that their perceptions of health and illness can be widely different. Such variations, if they are significant, add strength to the arguments supporting the need to relate quality to users' requirements. The following discussion draws upon Helman (1990) in detailing variations in health-illness beliefs and sub-cultural variations in health care provision.

HETEROGENEITY IN HEALTH CARE BELIEFS AND PRACTICES

Some of the doubt that user requirement and purchaser specification are not absolutely congruent arises from anthropological and sociological studies on cultural variations in health-illness and medicine beliefs. These are to be found, as Helman observes, across and within all communities of the UK. For example, he gives accounts of differing perceptions of anatomy, physiology, bodily functioning and standards of "beauty", and of "illness" and "health".

The variation in health-illness perception is matched by variations in medical treatment and therapy: Helman offers a classification of "medical subcultures" and lists over sixty kinds of healer in the UK. Clearly, there are a wide range of "therapeutic options" available to someone who seeks health care outside of the NHS. However, many of the healers listed by Helman would not find their services offered by the NHS since their practice is regarded as "quackery" (e.g. herbalists), and applications to offer their services would probably be met with scepticism.

We cannot claim, however, that "scientific medicine" - the dominant form of medicine in the NHS - is immune from sub-cultural variations. It is decidedly not homogenous. Helman provides evidence of medical and paramedical professional differences of perceptions of health, illness, treatment, competence, jargon, hierarchy and organisation. He also cites differences in drug prescribing and diagnosis both within the UK and internationally. The Conservative Government made a similar observation in its White Paper "Working For Patients" (HMSO, 1989), in referring to "wide variations" in drug prescribing by GPs, and "twenty-fold variations" in referrals to hospital across the UK. Here there is an indication of heterogeneity which may or may not be a response to differing demand by UK communities. This diversity appears to be rejected by the Government which is seeking uniformity in high quality health care provision, again implying a belief in some form of universal criteria.

The ambiguity of "scientific medicine" is deepened when pondering the finding that "many" orthodox (i.e. NHS scientific) doctors are practising some form of alternative or complementary medicine (Helman, 1990). This "alternative" practice occurs "outside" the formal boundaries of the NHS, implying a need to keep "unscientific" medical practices at arms length from the pure scientific medicine commonly practised.

This is not to say that *every* kind of alternative therapy is rejected. For example, the NHS formally offers homeopathic medicine which is fundamentally antithetical to scientific medicine. Yet to practice in an NHS homeopathic hospital, doctors must also be qualified and registered scientific doctors. The use by "scientific" practitioners of homeopathy and of informal "alternative" medicine suggests a suspension of belief in the rationality of scientific medicine in order to practice "unscientifically". Alternatively, justification might be sought in the use of the well known "placebo effect" as an explanation of any therapeutic effects of homeopathic practices. Such an explanation accords with the rationality of scientific medicine and thus reduces the dissonance which might otherwise be felt.

It has been argued that there are variations in health-illness belief and medical practice in the UK, and within the NHS. These variations have to be accounted for if a formal specification of NHS services is to meet user requirements. While medical practice in the NHS may have an informal component that is flexibly able to meet some requirements outside existing specifications, this informal practice should be open to questions about its legitimacy, validity, desirability and equity in provision. The possibility of considering these issues is further confounded by the unequal power relations which exist in the provider-purchaser-user relationship. This is the subject of the next section.

POWER RELATIONS BETWEEN USERS AND THE NHS

Several authors discuss the relations between medicine and society, and doctor and patient (see for example Parsons, 1951; Zola, 1972; and Patrick and Scambler, 1986). Another, particularly useful account is given by Hillier (1986) who provides a synthesis of several perspectives on "medicine as social control". In this analysis the influence that medicine has in society is described as deriving from its role in legitimising illness.

There are other roles which Hillier perceives medicine fulfilling, many of which serve to reinforce the powerful position held by medical science. For example, the defining and creation of new areas of medicine (medicalisation) falls to medicine, as does the capacity to medicalise normal lifestyles, e.g. the sale of vitamin pills. Clearly, Hillier is concerned with many of the negative effects of medical influence, and a comment concerning iatrogenisis (e.g. the creation of "dependency" as a consequence of medical activities and definitions of health and illness) bears witness to these detrimental influences.

These are by no means the only witnesses to the influence and power of medicine. Giddens (1991) refers to the "disembedding" of people through the need to trust professionals more generally, a point that is reflected in Hillier's concern about "power" given over to medical staff members who seek and receive "professional" status. This creates an inequity between patients and medical professionals who are perceived to be both knowledgeable and powerful whilst the patient is ignorant and weak.

The result of this unequal relationship is that the user is not in a position to readily challenge professionals to justify their actions. No wonder, then, that "advocacy" assumes an important role in empowering users, in person or by proxy, in the NHS. Such schemes as those organised by MIND or other self-help groups are discussed by Winn (1990). However, advocacy of this kind remains limited in scope and does not address fundamental problems. For example, in a three volume report to the Department of Health by Normand (1991) there is no mention of fully participative communication with users by NHS professions. The user is therefore in danger of being marginalised by paternalist NHS authorities who "know best", and whose position is recognised as authoritative by the user. Despite increasing conflicts as health care decisions are challenged through the courts by users, the user is still subordinate to the professional and in danger of further subjugation with the separation of purchasing and provision.

DIALOGUE AND THE NHS — THE POTENTIAL FOR QUALITY

The argument so far has criticised the current model of the NHS for its ambiguous concept of quality, for inadequately accounting for differences of health-illness and medicinal beliefs inside and outside of the NHS, and for failing to consider the effects of power in subjugating and dominating the user.

An alternative approach to quality in the NHS can now be considered which is ideologically distinct from those mentioned earlier. The method proposed focuses on the user as an equal and legitimate judge of quality, and will accommodate a diversity of perspectives. This approach is one of generating dialogue based upon requirements for "communicative competence" and "ideal speech" (Habermas, 1984). In identifying the need for an "ideal speech situation", Habermas recognises the factors preventing a "true" dialogue from occurring: power relations, differing beliefs, differing perceptions, differing values, etc. The call for "communicative competence" provides the minimum requirements in order that such barriers to "ideal speech" may be removed. Fairtlough (1989) states that the works of Habermas "provide a theoretical underpinning by describing what is *logically* necessary for reaching understanding between people, or, in other words, for excellent communication" (1989: 409).

It is worth considering Fairtlough's detailed explanation of Habermas's work, since it provides a useful insight into the application of the ideas in an industrial setting, which may be transferable to the NHS. There are five aspects of importance in generating an arena for dialogue, as follows:

- First, the actors in the situation have to be ready to discuss *objective matters* in a manner which, at least to some extent, follows the practice of natural science, basing their arguments on the agreement of observers who have investigated factual situations and have built theoretical models to explain them. Actors have to be ready to reject these models if they fail to account for observations or if they are superseded by simpler or more comprehensive models or by ones which have greater predictive capability.
- Second, these actors have to be ready to discuss *matters of right and wrong judged by reference to universal norms*. The norms themselves are open to challenge and (as in the case of factual matters) are, in the end, dependent on a consensus among those who have investigated the consistency, coherence, and universality of the set of norms which relate to these actions. Debate on norms is also dependent on the ability of the actors in the situation to achieve mutual understanding on ethical matters.
- Third, the *authenticity and sincerity* of actors involved in reaching mutual understanding must be open to confirmation. Again, the consensus of those who have considered the claims of sincerity (implicit or explicit) by relevant actors, using criteria of consistency and coherence, are the way in which the confirmation can be obtained.
- Fourth, not only must *standards and judgements* in all of the above three areas be open to criticism, but *agreement between those involved* must be actively sought. All three kinds of claim need to be taken into account together, i.e., claims to accuracy and truth in objective matters, to coherence and universality in normative matters, and to authenticity and sincerity on subjective expressions.

- Finally, the process of reaching mutual understanding should be the *co-operative negotiation* of common definitions of the situation, taking into account the possibility that factual, normative, and subjective aspects may all need common definition.

(Fairtlough 1989: 409-410, emphases added)

Under these conditions dialogue would offer the users of the NHS the opportunity to challenge and seek meaningful justification for the decisions that are made by the purchasers and providers of NHS services. Indeed, this is the only way that users can know at the time decisions are taken that the *investment* of resources, meaning taxpayers money *and* less tangible sacrifices by staff, patients and others, will produce services that are likely to meet their requirements. Simultaneously, the purchasers and the providers can challenge the users' expectations.

What is emerging from this discussion is the concept of an arena in which there is a continuous trial, without adversaries, and in which every participant is counsel, judge and jury, speaking and listening as equals. This is an ideal, but Fairtlough (1989) comments that he "has been surprised by what can be achieved in a business setting, which might not be regarded by many people as the easiest place to achieve communication of this kind" (Fairtlough, 1989: 410).

Clearly, the conditions of ideal speech and communicative competence cannot be employed simply through a statement of the necessary preconditions. There needs to be some method(s) for facilitating meetings in which there is a commitment to dialogue but where participants are drawn from a range of settings both within and outside of the NHS. Fairtlough has successfully utilised a number of "systems methods" within an organisation, and we intend to draw upon a framework of such systems methods in our practical research, currently being piloted in Sheffield. The interested reader might find Flood and Jackson (1991) or Jackson (1991) useful introductions to the framework we propose to use.

The pilot project in Sheffield involves the Royal Sheffield Institution for Blind people, Trent Regional Health Authority, Sheffield's Community Health Council, a University research team and, when commitment can be gained, Sheffield Health Authority and/or other purchasers. It is looking at the difficulties in establishing dialogue on quality in the services affecting blind people in Sheffield. Practical difficulties which have been identified include gaining commitments, time tabling, representation and participation, "fixed" constraints, difficulties with communication, and the effects of coercion. Other difficulties may be identified in the course of dialogue, and those listed above will be discussed below.

THE NEED FOR COMMITMENT — A NEW QUALITY IDEOLOGY

Fairtlough (1989) states that commitment to and belief in dialogue as a means to facilitate problem solving is an ideological essential. In a quality dialogue in the NHS there must be a similar ideological commitment. Indeed, involvement in dialogue means that NHS professionals would be committing themselves to the possibility of change when consensus is achieved. This is a new quality ideology, substantially different from the other ideologies of quality mentioned previously.

TIMETABLE

Fairtlough (1989) contends that participants must accept an abbreviated process for urgent issues because time is not infinitely available. He makes the practical suggestion that systems methods may be employed to assess the potential for approximating to an ideal speech situation in order that the scope for abbreviation can be determined. At the same time, the relative importance of the elements leading to ideal speech can be discussed. Clearly, Fairtlough is advocating debate about debate in which formulae may be derived which will guide the future handling of urgent issues. In Sheffield the dialogue may produce a near infinite agenda, but those who are in the dialogue would have the opportunity to suggest priorities and modifications, or could even justify terminating it.

REPRESENTATION AND PARTICIPATION

Clearly there are issues of representation and participation that have to be resolved. There will be many dialogues, and the users who participate at an appointed time and place can only be a sample. However, this is not the only difficulty associated with representation. We need to ask: what is the nature and status of their representation? Will users undertake something akin to jury service? Or voluntary service? Will they be randomly selected from the population? It is accepted that representation can never be total, and that representativeness of the groups present will be subject to dialogue. In this way participants may seek improvements in the form and content of their representation. In Sheffield, the RSIB are assisting in obtaining a self-selecting group of blind people as participants in the dialogue. There will be assistance in facilitation from the Community Health Council and Trent Regional Health Authority, but the purchaser and provider representation have yet to be determined.

STAKEHOLDER CONSTRAINTS

In the light of new understandings and information generated through the process, stakeholders may wish to modify their proposed actions but may be unable to do so due to external constraints. It is at this point that dialogue offers the opportunity for stakeholders to develop more realistic expectations, or to explore new, possibly more radical, alternatives. However, we must acknowledge that in some circumstances such a possibility may not arise due to the problems associated with unequal relationships within the health care system.

An interesting discussion of the capacity for stakeholder participation through campaigning is given by Midgley (1992). Here, the focus is on an alternative arena in which stakeholders can address issues outside of the forum in which power relations act to prevent the stakeholders' legitimate influence on decision making. An example might be where those negatively affected by a particular drug have grouped together to seek legal assistance in gaining recognition of their grievance.

DIFFICULTIES WITH COMMUNICATIONS

Normand (1991, volume 3), in reporting on quality issues to the Department of Health, noted several comments on the desirability of interdisciplinary communication in the NHS (for example, Working Paper No 6 of *Working For Patients*, H.M.S.O., 1989). He found that there is literary evidence of many interdisciplinary communications in the United States, whilst only one account could be found in the UK.

This major observation is the last comment of Normand's literature review, but it is not included in the executive summary. This may have resulted in the Department of Health attaching little importance to the issue. Our argument suggests that such an omission is not legitimate, and that dialogue *is* required in order that issues surrounding the quality of health care provision may be aired. Furthermore, such dialogue should not exclude users as is implied by Normand's focus on "interdisciplinary communications". Given the possibility of a language gap between users and professionals, this may appear to be a tall order. Nevertheless, commitment to dialogue involving users as well as providers is essential.

COERCIVE RELATIONSHIPS

It could be argued that coercive power relations are rife in the NHS, which has many latent conflicts. These have been most publicly aired in the disagreements on the issue of the NHS reforms between the Government, the British Medical Association and the Royal College of Nursing. There has also been industrial action connected with this issue. Coercive conditions are antithetical to the conditions necessary for ideal speech. The turbulent coerciveness of the NHS must be overcome in order to facilitate dialogue. However, this must be handled carefully, since coercion of coercive elements simply perpetuates the difficulty in another area.

The only strategy available would appear to be one in which the situation is transformed from coercive to non-coercive. This may be done by the negotiation of territory in the NHS in which the ideological commitment to dialogue mentioned by Fairtlough (1989) is a condition of entry. Hence in Sheffield there will be a period of negotiation with purchasers and providers in which they may wish to protect their interests. Ordinarily, negotiation entails the use of power. Consensus therefore cannot reflect the "force of the better argument", but rather the "force of the better bargain". Bargaining over interests cannot necessarily, in practice, be excluded from a quality dialogue, but the distinction between negotiation and dialogue has to be borne in mind.

WAYS FORWARD — CREATING A NEW ARENA FOR DIALOGUE

The question still remains, how can a group of diverse people begin to communicate ideally and competently with each other, preferably within a year or two? It is more complicated when it is realised that these groups will not remain static since new individuals would be entering and leaving all the time. One approach that may offer some hope is that of a new form of advocacy, perhaps developed from some existing user organisation such as the Community Health Council. The advocates would be acting as interpreters and communicators, rather than as powerful negotiators. In the Sheffield pilot study, this role will be undertaken initially by the researchers. It may be that education and training could improve the competence of the speakers and increase the participants' understanding of the conditions necessary for the existence of the arena.

Finally, the tripartite agreement that would form the "new arena" in the NHS might be more easily obtained by commencing with a discussion of the possible content of the agenda. This might help to generate a "formula" agenda which could be utilised in future debates. By delineating some common boundary or reference point, the ability of the participants to relate with one another according to Habermasian ideals may be enhanced.

Finally, there is a necessity that some means be available of resolving the difficulties that emerge from the dialogue. Dialogue would be discouraged by the unhappy experience of handling issues beyond the abilities of stakeholders. Any means to overcome these difficulties must be contextually determined and ratified by the participants. We anticipate that one outcome of our research will be the description of such means.

CONCLUSION

It has been shown that quality is an increasingly important issue within the National Health Service. A number of definitions of "quality" have been considered, together with questions related to the process of determining who should judge quality. A model was proposed for the implementation of a tripartite dialogue involving NHS providers, purchasers and users. Several difficulties likely to be encountered were also discussed. Finally, mention was made of a project in which the ideas contained in this paper will be put to practice.

REFERENCES

BSI 1987. *BS 5750: British Standard for assuring quality.* British Standards Institute: Milton Keynes.

Donabedian, A. 1980. *The definition of quality and approaches to its assessment.* Ann Arbor: Michigan.

Department of Trade and Industry. 1991. *Total Quality Management.* Department of Trade and Industry, PUB260: London.

Fairtlough, G. 1989. Systems practice from the start: some experiences in a biotechnology company *Systems Practice.* **Vol. 2.** No. 4. 397-412.

Flood, R and Jackson, M. 1991. *Creative problem solving: Total Systems Intervention.* John Wiley: Chichester.

Giddens, A. 1991. *Modernity and self identity.* Polity Press: Cambridge.

Habermas J. 1984. *The theory of communicative action vol.1* (translated by T. McCarthy). Heinemann: London

Helman, C. 1990. *Culture, health and illness.* Wright: London.

Hillier, S. M. 1986. Medicine and Social Control In Patrick, D. and Scambler, G. (eds.). 1986. *Sociology as applied to medicine.* Bailliere Tindall: London.

HMSO. 1989. *Working for Patients.* HMSO: London.

Jackson, M.C. 1991. *Systems Methodology for the Management Sciences.* Plenum: New York.

Maxwell, R. 1984. Quality assessment in health *British Medical Journal.* **Vol. 289.** 1470-1472.

Maynard, A. 1992. *Competition in Health Care: Whatever Happened to the Government Health Reforms?* Dept. of Social Policy and Professional Studies: University of Hull.

Midgley, G. 1992. Power and languages of co-operation: a critical systems perspective In *Systemica '92: 1ra. Conferencia Internacional de Trabajo del Instituto Andino de Systemas (IAS),* held on 23-28 August 1992.

Munro-Faure, L & Munro-Faure, M. 1992. *Implementing Total Quality Management.* Pitman: London.

Normand, C. 1991. *Clinical audit in professions allied to medicine and related therapy professions: Report to the Department of Health.* Health and health care research unit: Belfast.

Oakland, J. 1989. *Total quality management.* Heinemann: Oxford.

Parsons, T. 1951. *The Social System.* Routledge & Kegan Paul: London

Patrick, D. and Scambler, G. (eds.) 1986. *Sociology as applied to medicine.* Bailliere Tindall: London.

Rainbow. 1991. *Using information in managing the nursing resource.* Greenhalgh & Company Ltd: Macclesfield.

Shaw, C. 1986. *Quality assurance, what the colleges are doing.* King Edwards hospital fund: London.

Taguchi, G. 1979. *Introduction to off-line quality control.* Central Japan Quality Control Association: Magaya, Japan.

Winn, L. (ed.). 1990. *Power to the people.* Kings Fund Centre: London.

Zola, I. K. 1972. Medicine as an institution of social control *Sociological Review.* **Vol. 20.** No. 4. 487-509.

13 Quantifying Quality — Measuring Quality in the Provision of Health Care

PAUL KIND[1], BRENDA LEESE[1], IAN CAMERON[2] & JENNIE CARPENTER[3]

[1]Centre for Health Economics, University of York
[2]Department of Public Health Medicine, Leeds Health Authority
[3]North Yorkshire Health Authority

INTRODUCTION

General Practitioners (GPs) are becoming increasingly important players in the emerging health care market place. This enhanced role is shared by all GPs and is not restricted to fundholders with their additional financial leverage. They now have a key role in determining contract standards and monitoring service delivery, and the nature of their clinical practice enables them to directly influence referral patterns. Purchasing authorities now increasingly look to GPs for observation and comment on the quality and quantity of services available from local provider units, whereas in the past such opinion was seldom sought. Even if the views of GPs were sought, it is doubtful whether they were given any serious consideration. Now that GPs have a more pivotal role within the reformed NHS, their opinions are more likely to affect change. The unique agency relationship in which the GP acts on behalf the patient enhances the need to utilise these views to the full. The development of a low-cost survey method which enables the views of GPs to be represented, would seem therefore, to afford a significant advance over past practice. The results obtained from such a survey are described in this chapter.

NUMERIC METHODS

Problems with arbitrary scores

Several reports have appeared in the literature (Donald and Berman: 1989; Walker, Griffiths and Leon: 1991; White, Williams and Richards: 1991; Madden: 1985; Robb and Johnston: 1991; Sutton et al: 1987; Hicks and Baker: 1991 and Bowling et al:

Managerial Issues in the Reformed NHS. Edited by M.Malek, P.Vacani, J.Rasquinha & P.Davey
© 1993 John Wiley & Sons Ltd

1991) giving details of surveys of GP perceptions of local service provision. Whilst these reports represent an important source of information regarding the state of play at a single point in time, they are less helpful in providing a means of monitoring the effects of any changes which may result. The interpretation of such data is often difficult, since the results are based on distributions of responses, rather than a summary statistic or index. For example, Table 1 shows hypothetical survey data, which relates to 3 hospital services, rated on a 4 point category scale from "outstanding" to "poor". All 3 services have a combined rating of 70% for the 2 higher categories. Service B dominates service A if only 'outstanding' ratings are taken into account. On the other hand service C outperforms both A and B on this basis. What is to be made, however, of the higher proportions of 'poor' ratings given to service C? What weight should be attached to these data? How overall, would results for service C be assessed? How would the services be ranked one against another?

Table 1. Hypothetical Survey Data

Service	Rating			
	Outstanding	Good	Satisfactory	Poor
A	20%	50%	20%	10%
B	50%	20%	20%	10%
C	60%	10%	10%	20%

Differences in the distribution of scores makes it difficult to compare services. The need for a simpler method seems clear, and this paper reports one technique for achieving this. The basis of the method is not new, since its origins can be traced back to work in experimental psychology of nearly 70 years ago (Thurstone: 1927). The application of methods for scaling categorical data with the intention of deriving a weighted quality index, however, appears not to have been previously attempted.

Derivation of the Quality Index

Thurstone's (1927) work on paired comparisons and category rating methods has long been used to derive quantitative measures of subjective opinion. These techniques have formed part of the psychometric researcher's tool kit ever since their original publication nearly 70 years ago. More recently Torgerson (1958) described a categorical scaling model linked to this earlier work. Before presenting the results of the survey, the stages involved in computing values for a Quality Index according to this basic model will be described.

Assume for a moment that subjective judgements about quality of service reflect an underlying continuum that is represented by a line. Good quality, as a characteristic of health authority services, is located towards one end of the line, and poor quality is located towards the opposite end. Arranged along the line are a number of boundaries which define intervals or categories (Figure 1).

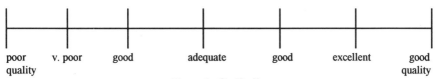

| poor | v. poor | good | adequate | good | excellent | good |
| quality | | | | | | quality |

Figure 1. Quality line

Torgerson defines a procedure for deriving arithmetic values for the category boundaries, thereby allowing estimates to be made of the scale values of items located along the line. By utilising information about the frequency with which observers (in this case GPs) place services in each of the categories, it is possible to calculate values for the category boundaries, and from these to estimate values for the services themselves.

In summary, Torgerson's model postulates that:

- an individual's psychological continuum (in this case perceived quality of service) can be divided into a finite series of ordered categories;
- because of many factors, including experimental error and subject performance, the boundary between adjacent categories varies and gives rise to a normal distribution around a mean location;
- different category boundaries may have different means and distributions;
- a subject will place an item (e.g. hospital service) below a given category boundary when the value of that item on the quality continuum is lower than the value of that category boundary.

The computational steps are simple and are demonstrated here using the ratings for diagnostic services produced by 112 GPs who rated 7 diagnostic services on a scale from 1 to 5 (excellent to very poor). These ratings are summarised in Table 2 which shows the basic frequency matrix F.

Table 2. Frequency Matrix F — Diagnostic Services

| (rank) | Quality Rating | | | | | |
	excellent	good	adequate	poor	very poor	weighted row sum
Microbiology (2)	43	65	4	0	0	185
Histopathology (4.5)	36	71	4	0	0	190
Biochemistry (4.5)	40	66	6	0	0	190
Haemotology (3)	43	61	8	0	0	189
Radiology (6)	14	47	38	10	3	277
Ultrasound (7)	11	35	30	25	11	326
Nuclear Medicine (1)	24	59	14	0	0	184

This relatively simple matrix contains a wealth of information:

- The form of the distribution of categories assigned to each state.

Microbiology, for example, has a very compact distribution with (43+65)/112 respondents rating in categories 1+2 (excellent and very good). By comparison, ultrasound ratings appear throughout the full range from excellent to very poor.
- The overall rank of the states.

The weighted row sum is given in the final column. This is computed by multiplying each Fij element by its corresponding category (1 = excellent .... 5 = very poor), across each row (e.g. for microbiology = 43x1 + 65x2 + 4x3 = 185). On the basis of these totals, nuclear medicine and ultrasound would be placed at the top and bottom of the quality rankings.

The information in the F matrix can be interpreted as probabilities rather than frequencies. Hence in this sample of GPs the probability of microbiology receiving an excellent rating was 43/112 (0.38). All elements in the F matrix are now converted into their corresponding probabilities. The next stage in deriving the Quality Index involves constructing a cumulative probability matrix by summing across rows (Table 3). For example, microbiology, has a probability of an excellent rating of 43/112 (0.38), a probability of a good rating of 65/112 (0.58) and a probability of an adequate rating of 4/112 (0.04). Since all general practitioners had rated microbiology in the first three categories all 'votes' had been exhausted at this point. The probability of placing microbiology in category 3 or higher is 1.0 and remains so across all remaining elements in that row. The last column (5 in this example) will always have a probability of 1.0, and is discarded for the remaining stages of the computation.

Table 3: P-Matrix (Cumulative Probabilities)

	Quality Rating Category				
	1	2	3	4	5
Microbiology	0.38	0.96	1.00	1.00	1.00
Histopathology	0.32	0.96	1.00	1.00	1.00
Biochemistry	0.36	0.95	1.00	1.00	1.00
Haematology	0.38	0.93	1.00	1.00	1.00
Radiology	0.13	0.54	0.88	0.97	1.00
Ultrasound	0.10	0.41	0.68	0.90	1.00
Nuclear Medicine	0.25	0.86	1.00	1.00	1.00

The probabilities in the P-matrix are converted, using standard tables, into corresponding z-scores based on the unit normal distribution (Table 4). Where there are probabilities of 0 or 1, indicating perfect certainty in predicting categories, these elements are flagged as missing data since they strictly yield z-scores of infinity. In the transformed matrix these are shown as **.

Table 4. Z Matrix (z-scores based on the P-Matrix)

Microbiology	-0.29	1.80	**	**
Histopathology	-0.46	1.80	**	**
Biochemistry	-0.37	1.61	**	**
Haematology	-0.29	1.47	**	**
Radiology	-1.15	0.11	1.19	1.93
Ultrasound	-1.29	-0.23	0.46	1.29
Nuclear Medicine	-0.68	1.06	**	**

Such incomplete matrices are commonplace in practical settings and a variety of algorithms have been proposed in order to overcome the problem of estimating category boundaries and scale values. Torgerson describes one such procedure based on the average differences between categories. Hence for microbiology the absolute difference between the first and second columns (in matrix notation [3] $z(1,1) - z(1,2)$ [3]) is -0.29 - 1.80 = 2.09. (Table 5).

Table 5. Absolute Differences

	z (i,1) - z(i,2)	z(i,2) - z(i,3)	z(i,3 - z(i,4)	z(i,4) - z(i,5)
Microbiology	2.10	**	**	**
Histopatholgy	2.25	**	**	**
Biochemistry	1.98	**	**	**
Haematology	1.76	**	**	**
Radiology	1.26	1.08	0.74	0.93
Ultrasound	1.07	0.69	0.83	0.29
Nuclear Medicine	1.74	**	**	**
mean column totals	**1.74**	**0.89**	**0.79**	**0.61**
category boundary	**0.000**	**1.74**	**2.63**	**3.41**

(rounding in the print routines used to display these figures means that some elements may have slight arithmetic differences).

The lowest category boundary is set to zero, and successive boundaries are generated by accumulating the average differences. The scale values are given by computing the mean difference between category boundary scores and the corresponding elements in the Z-matrix.

The calculation for microbiology is $(0.0 + 0.29) + (1.74 - 1.80) = (0.23 / 2)$ since all other elements are missing values, and this yields a mean of 0.115 (the unadjusted score for microbiology) (Table 6).

Table 6. Scale Values

Service	Unadjusted Score	Transformed Score
Microbiology	0.155	0.697
Histopathology	0.197	0.687
Biochemistry	0.246	0.681
Haematology	0.283	0.676
Nuclear Medicine	0.679	0.627
Radiology	1.420	0.535
Ultrasound	1.882	0.478

A further modification has been introduced in deriving these scale values. There exist two theoretical extremes to the pattern of quality ratings. All ratings could be in category 1 (excellent) or in category 5 (very poor). By superimposing these two additional sets of quality ratings it is possible to establish the proportion of the theoretical maximum quality score for each of the services. The final stage in calculating quality scores using the Torgerson algorithm is shown in the last column. In this case the raw score for microbiology of 0.115 becomes 0.697, or 69.7% of the theoretical maximum.

It is interesting to compare the ranks of the weighted Quality Index with the ranks shown in the F-matrix (Table 2). Nuclear Medicine now drops to 5th, and is replaced in 1st. position by Microbiology, which had received a similar weighted row sum in the F-matrix. The tie between Histopathology and Biochemistry is broken by the ranked Quality Index, although a difference of 0.006 is probably insufficient to clearly distinguish between services.

METHODS

The survey

Although the model has been applied in the assessment of quality in more than one Health Authority, the results from only one of these studies are reported here. A postal questionnaire was sent to each of 145 GPs in 46 practices. Four weeks were allowed for return of the questionnaires, after which reminders were sent to the non-respondents. Two weeks later, practice managers were telephoned to ask them to encourage the remaining non-responders to complete the questionnaire. The questionnaire had been discussed with GP and consultant representatives before circulation, and covered five topics. The opening section asked for some details about the respondent and her or his practice. A second section listed hospital services (n=31), community services (n=19) and diagnostic services (n=7) available to district residents and asked general practitioners to give each service a general quality rating on a scale of 1 = excellent, 2 = good, 3 = adequate, 4 = poor, 5 = very poor, 6 = insufficient evidence to judge quality. Figure 1 shows an example page from the questionnaire. The final sections of the questionnaire recorded more detailed information regarding specific criteria used by GPs in evaluating the quality of services. Further questions were also included, asking GPs to identify those services in need of improvement.

Survey Response Rates

The questionnaire was returned by 112 out of a possible 145 GPs giving an overall response rate of 77%. There were also five specific refusals or letters in response and five questionnaires were returned too late for inclusion in the analysis, so that only 23 general practitioners failed to respond at all. Most of the respondents (70%) had been working in the area for 10 years or less, and their average age was 40.6 years. 38 (34%) worked in a training practice and 23 (20.5%) were female. There was no significant variation in response by partnership size and no other evidence that the non-responders were a selected group.

Quality Ratings for Hospital Services

Paediatrics stood out with virtually 100% of GPs giving it a rating of excellent or good, as shown in Table 7. Cardiology also had a high rating and there was then a group of specialties, including general medicine, general surgery, dermatology, rheumatology, diabetology with almost all good or adequate ratings. Only a quarter of GPs rated ophthalmology as excellent or good and only 10% so rated orthopaedics. Other poorly rated services included psycho-sexual counselling where, although only 78% of GPs felt able to rate this service, nearly 74% rated it poor or very poor. Services for the younger disabled were also rated as poor or very poor by half of the 73 GPs rating it. The rating given to the pain clinic was interesting as equal proportions of GPs rated it excellent/good, adequate and poor/very poor. There were some services that a majority of GPs felt unable to rate; services for HIV/AIDS sufferers were rated only by a third of GPs of whom only 30% rated it excellent or good.

Quality Index values for hospital services are listed in Table 8. As is to be expected, the values reflect the general pattern of ratings reported above, with paediatrics scoring very highly. Cardiology, including general medicine with related specialties, and general surgery, have Quality Index values of 60% or above. The poor/very poor ratings given to psychosexual counselling are reflected in the relatively low Quality Index of 32%. The value of 42% achieved by orthopaedics is only about half that attained by paediatrics.

Table 7. Quality Ratings Given by General Practitioners for Hospital Specialties

Specialty/Service	Frequency of rating in each quality category					Number of GPs giving a rating of 1-5
	1	2	3	4	5	
General Medicine	17	72	21	2	0	112
General Surgery	15	71	23	3	0	112
Paediatrics	74	37	1	0	0	112
Obstetrics	10	62	28	12	0	112
Gynaecology	4	32	49	26	1	112
Geriatric Services	5	35	46	22	4	112
Orthopaedics	2	10	36	51	13	112
Psychiatry	2	32	58	12	5	109
Psychogeriatrics	17	48	28	11	1	105
Accident & Emergency	11	72	24	2	0	109
Rheumatology	14	69	26	2	0	111
Dermatology	16	78	18	0	0	112
Paediatric Surgery	5	24	19	7	3	58*
Renal Medicine	9	41	20	3	1	74*
Neurology	7	47	45	8	0	107
Genito-Urinary Med	7	55	33	9	1	105
Oncology	13	46	24	7	2	92*
Chest Medicine	19	71	16	3	1	110
Ophthalmology	4	24	43	36	4	111
HIV/AIDS Services	1	10	16	8	2	37*
Younger Disabled	3	10	24	27	9	73*
Gastroenterology	2	39	57	12	2	112
Ear, Nose & Throat	8	65	32	6	0	111
Urology	13	59	27	11	0	110
Plastic Surgery	7	32	31	18	2	90*
Cardiology	35	57	18	2	0	112
Cardiac Surgery	11	28	33	17	1	90*
Diabetes	25	55	28	4	0	112
Child & Adolescent Psychiatry	6	52	29	4	0	91*
Psychosexual Counselling	0	3	20	28	36	87*
Pain Clinic	4	35	35	34	3	111

Ratings: 1 = excellent, 2 = good, 3 = adequate, 4 = poor, 5 = very poor.

Note: Table 1 lists the number of GPs who rated each specialty, in each of the five quality categories. The total number of GPs who rated the service is given in the final column of this table. Where more than 10% of GPs indicated that they had insufficient evidence to give a rating of quality, then this total is marked by the symbol *.

Table 8: Quality Index Values for Hospital Specialties

Rank	Hospital Specialty/Service	Standardised Quality Index
1	Paediatrics	0.797
2	Cardiology	0.656
3	General Medicine	0.631
4	Dermatology	0.626
5	Rheumatology	0.620
6	Diabetes	0.619
7	General Surgery	0.617
8	Accident & Emergency	0.616
9	Chest Medicine	0.609
10	Renal Medicine	0.579*
11.5	Ear, Nose & Throat Surgery	0.577
11.5	Child & Adolescent Psychiatry	0.577*
13	Urology	0.575
14	Psychogeriatrics	0.571
15	Obstetrics	0.566
16	Oncology	0.564*
17	Genito-Urinary Medicine	0.557
18	Neurology	0.553
19	Cardiac Surgery	0.540*
20	Paediatric Surgery	0.522*
21	Plastic Surgery	0.521*
22.5	Gastroenterology	0.510
22.5	Gynaecology	0.510
24	Medicine for the Elderly	0.500
25	Pain Clinic	0.491
26	Psychiatry	0.489
27	HIV/AIDS Services	0.479*
28	Ophthalmology	0.477
29	Younger Disabled	0.442*
30	Orthopaedics	0.416
31	Psychosexual Counselling	0.318*

(Derivation of the Standardised Quality Index from the Quality Ratings is given in the text.)

Quality Ratings for Community Services

Table 9 shows ratings for 19 community services. Terminal care provided by the Hospice received over 90% excellent or good ratings, terminal care in the community had 75% excellent or good ratings; in contrast, terminal care in hospital had only 22% excellent or good ratings. District nursing services and community midwifery were rated excellent or good by over 65% of GPs, whereas community child health, mental health services and family planning were only seen as adequate by the majority of GPs.

Table 9. Quality Ratings Given by General Practitioners for Community Services

Community Service	Frequency rating in each quality category					Number of GPs giving a rating of 1-5
	1	2	3	4	5	
Mental Handicap Services	0	18	44	13	3	78*
Terminal Care Hospice	55	39	4	5	0	103
Terminal Care Hospital	3	19	49	22	5	98*
Terminal Care Community	30	51	21	4	1	107
Health Visiting	10	32	46	20	3	111
District Nursing	27	44	31	9	0	111
Community Midwifery	31	44	24	8	4	111
Community Child Health	1	23	49	1	11	85*
Family Planning	7	30	49	5	2	93*
Disability & Rehabilitation	1	8	26	35	8	78*
Physiotherapy	7	22	38	37	5	109
Occupational Therapy	2	22	35	22	5	86*
Dietetics	3	39	48	13	2	105
Chiropody	2	17	35	40	11	105
Speech Therapy	5	31	38	18	6	98*
Alcohol & Drug Abuse	1	18	30	25	13	87*
Audiology	15	46	42	2	1	106*
Appliances - Hospital	4	29	34	16	2	85*
Appliances - Joint Equipment	3	21	27	14	0	65*

Ratings: 1 = excellent, 2 = good, 3 = adequate, 4 = poor, 5 = very poor.

Note: This table lists the number of GPs who rated each specialty, in each of the five quality categories. The total number of GPs who rated the service is given in the final column of this table. Where more than 10% of GPs indicated that they had insufficient evidence to give a rating of quality, then this total is marked by the symbol *.

Disability and rehabilitation services were poorly rated, with 35 of the 78 GPs able to assess these services giving a poor or very poor rating. Chiropody and services for alcohol and drug misusers were also rated poorly, with just under 50% of GPs rating them poor or very poor.

The Quality Index values for community services are given in Table 10. Half have values of around 50% or lower.   Hospice-based terminal care scores highly by comparison with most other services in this group.

Scoring below 50% of the theoretical maximum are physiotherapy, hospital terminal care, occupational therapy, chiropody, alcohol and drug misuse services, and disability and rehabilitation services.

Table 10. Quality Index Values for Community Services

Rank	Community Service	Standardised Quality Index
1	Terminal Care - Hospice	0.687
2	Terminal Care - Community	0.620
3	District Nursing	0.602
4	Audiology	0.596*
5	Community Midwifery	0.582
6	Family Planning	0.546*
7	Health Visiting	0.525
8	Dietetics	0.522
9	Appliances - Hospital	0.517*
10.5	Appliances - Joint Equipment	0.507*
10.5	Community Child Health	0.507*
12	Speech Therapy	0.499*
13	Mental Handicap Services	0.495*
14	Physiotherapy	0.486
15	Terminal Care - Hospital	0.479*
16	Occupational Therapy	0.475*
17	Chiropody	0.438
18	Alcohol & Drug Abuse	0.433*
19	Disability & Rehabilitation	0.420*

Ranked Quality Index Values

Table 11 shows all services, including Diagnostic Services, ranked by their Quality Index divided into four quartile bands. The singular pattern of ratings for paediatrics resulted in a high Quality Index value which appears much greater than that of all other services.

Table 11. All Services Ranked by Quality Index Score Divided into Four Quartiles

Rank	Service	Standardised Quality Index
1	Paediatrics	0.797
2	Microbiology	0.697
3.5	Terminal Care - Hospice	0.687
3.5	Histopathology	0.687
5	Biochemistry	0.681
6	Haematology	0.676
7	Cardiology	0.656
8	General Medicine	0.631
9	Nuclear Medicine	0.627*
10	Dermatology	0.626
11.5	Terminal Care - Community	0.620
11.5	Rheumatology	0.620
13	Diabetes	0.619
14	General Surgery	0.617
15	Accident & Emergency	0.616
16	Chest Medicine	0.609
17	District Nursing	0.602
18	Audiology	0.596*
19	Community Midwifery	0.582
20	Renal Medicine	0.579*
21.5	Ear, Nose & Throat Surgery	0.577
21.5	Child & Adolescent Psychiatry	0.577*
23	Urology	0.575
24	Psychogeriatrics	0.571
25	Obstetrics	0.566
26	Oncology	0.564*
27	Genito-Urinary Medicine	0.557
28	Neurology	0.553

29	Family Planning	0.546*
30	Cardiac Surgery	0.540*
31	Radiology	0.535
32	Health Visiting	0.525
33.5	Dietetics	0.522
33.5	Paediatric Surgery	0.522*
35	Plastic Surgery	0.521*
36	Appliances - Hospital	0.517*
37.5	Gastroenterology	0.510
37.5	Gynaecology	0.510
39.5	Appliances - Joint Equipment	0.507*
39.5	Community Child Health	0.507*
41	Medicine for the Elderly	0.500
42	Speech Therapy	0.499*
43	Mental Handicap Services	0.495*
44	Pain Clinic	0.491
45	Psychiatry	0.489
46	Physiotherapy	0.486
47.5	Terminal Care - Hospital	0.479*
47.5	HIV/AIDS Services	0.479*
49	Ultrasound	0.478
50	Opthalmology	0.477
51	Occupational therapy	0.475*
52	Younger Disabled	0.442*
53	Chiropody	0.438
54	Alcohol and Drug Abuse	0.433*
55	Disability and Rehabilitation	0.420*
56	Orthopaedics	0.416
57	Psychosexual Counselling	0.318*

The Quality Index for psychosexual counselling was the lowest, although this rating may be biased by the relatively large number of GPs who felt unable to assess the service quality owing to insufficient evidence. This argument may or may not bear close scrutiny, since other service areas, for example nuclear medicine, which some GPs also felt unable to assess, attracted higher ratings and hence, higher Quality Index scores.

DISCUSSION

Given the prevailing circumstances with contract and fundholding issues to the fore, the response rate of 77% must be regarded as excellent. There was a remarkable unanimity about which services were rated highly and which received poor ratings. The fact that so many general practitioners replied gives weight to the findings as being representative across the district.

Paediatrics received the highest standardised quality rating. Other services rated as of good quality were pathology, terminal care in the hospice, general medicine and related specialties, general surgery and accident and emergency services. Orthopaedics and ophthalmology were major hospital specialties rated as less good. Other services rated of less good quality were HIV/AIDS services, terminal care in hospital, ultrasound, chiropody, physiotherapy, younger disabled services, occupational therapy, disability and rehabilitation service, services for drug and alcohol misuse, and psychosexual counselling.

There were some services that many GPs felt they had insufficient evidence to rate overall. These included services for HIV/AIDS (rated by 37/112 GPs), services for the younger disabled (rated by 73/112 GPs) and paediatric surgery (rated by 58/112 GPs). This suggests that it would be useful to ensure that all GPs have some knowledge of how to access such services which are used relatively infrequently, particularly by smaller practices, so that patients within its catchment area receive the full range of services that the commissioning authority can offer to residents.

The results of this type of study should not be used in isolation. In a separate, but related part of this study, GPs were asked to choose 3 hospital and 3 community services which they felt were in need of improvement, and to record their reasons for their dissatisfaction. In the case of hospital services, GPs overwhelmingly nominated orthopaedics and ophthalmology as services in need of improvement - both of which scored poorly on the Quality Index. This type of study should be linked to discussion between GPs, consultants and managers, to ascertain the detail of any problems relating to services which are perceived as providing poor quality. Following such dialogue, and after any remedial action has been implemented, the same questionnaire-based system can be used to monitor the effects of any changes.

A standardised index of quality requires further testing as a management tool. The index gives only a broad indication of perceived quality and does not itself give an indication of the reasons behind particular ratings. The Quality Index could be used to measure changing views over time, or as a means of testing the impact of changes in service provision. If steps were taken to improve services with a low Quality Index, these changes ought to be reflected in an improved quality rating. GPs tend to remain in a specific practice over reasonably long periods of time, so that changes in the value of the Quality Index for specific services could be plotted against time, to provide a continually updated assessment of quality by a stable, expert, reference group. The index could also be used to compare services from different providers, particularly where GPs have a realistic choice. It could also be developed to test its potential more generally as a "performance indicator".

The presentation of data relating to perceived quality of service needs careful and sensitive handling. Simply showing a distribution of category ratings for example, has some merit in exposing the full range of information. However, such an approach harbours serious limitations, in that the relative importance of different categories remains unknown or is arbitrarily determined. Assigning increasing numeric values to adjacent categories is one way of reducing the complexity of the distributional data to a single index, but as has been shown in the worked example, it may lead to results which differ from those obtained by a less quixotic method of weighting. Whilst further detailed analysis of the data reported here may reveal the underlying structure which drives the assessment of quality, it is the final product of that process which is of most value to the health service manager. The relationship between the Quality Index and activity levels needs to be examined, as does the link between quality and outcomes. In the short-run the need is for a demonstration of the reliability of the methodology described here, and in particular the capacity to signal change when significant alteration to local services have been instituted.

In examining the reliability and validity of the Index it is important to demonstrate a positive relationship between quality ratings and other indicators of service quality. For example, external validation might be claimed if a correlation were to be demonstrated between Quality Index scores and a service performance indicator, such as waiting time. The reported study did not access such data. Some evidence of internal construct validity was achieved in that services nominated for improvement by GPs were typically those which had received low Quality Index scores. Further evidence of validity rests in the free-text responses made by GPs when completing their questionnaires. The overall consistency between GPs in their responses when rating services, lends weight to the argument that these data truly reflect GP assessment of quality, rather than merely recording some general measure of (dis)satisfaction.

Underlying the National Health Service reforms is the assumption that GPs will, in choosing secondary health care services, reflect their patients' wishes. This implies that GPs and patients share similar views on what constitutes a good quality service. If patients' views on the quality of local services were quantified using the methodology described here then a direct comparison could be made, and the extent to which services are similarly rated by GPs and patients alike can be tested empirically. However, focusing attention on the process of health care, and in particular on the perception of quality, may in the long run be shown as somewhat peripheral to the central task in evaluating services, since the main issue is not the quality of services, but their outcome. But that is, as they say, another story.

REFERENCES

Bowling, A., Jacobson, B., Southgate, L., Formby, J. General Practitioners' Views on Quality Specifications for "Outpatient Referrals and Care Contracts", British Medical Journal, 1991; 303: 292-294.

Donald, I.P. and Berman, P. Geriatric Outpatient Clinics - an audit of clinical action, transport and general practitioner views, Age and Ageing, 1989; 18: 253-257.

Hicks, N.R., Baker, I.A. General Practitioners' Opinions of Health Services Available to their Patients, British Medical Journal, 1991; 302: 991-993.

Madden, F.J.F., Analysis of Views of General Practitioners in Leicestershire on Chemotherapy, Clin. Radiol., 1985; 36: 663-664.

Robb, P.J. and Johnston, D. The Clinical Management of Otorrhea Following Grommet Insertion — a survey of otolaryngologists and general practitioners, Clinical Otolaryngology, 1991; 16: 367-370.

Sutton, P.P., Alexander, E.R., Russell, G. *et al.* Acute Asthma in the Grampian Region, 1976-85 - hospital admissions and GP survey, Thorax, 1987; 42: 733-734.

Thurstone, L.L. Method of paired comparisons for social values, Journal of Abnormal Social Psychology, 1927; 21: 384-400.

Torgerson, W.S. The Theory and Methods of Scaling, John Wiley, New York, 1958.

Walker, D.J., Griffiths, I.D. and Leon, C.M. Referrals to a Rheumatology Unit - an evaluation of the views of patients, general practitioners and consultants, Ann. Rheumatic Diseases, 1991; 50: 926-929.

White, P.M.B., Williams, H. and Richards, J. Survey of GP Attitudes to Microbiology Services, J. Clin. Path., 1991; 44: 615.

14 A Case Study of the Effectiveness of Management Training and Development in the NHS and Implications for Achieving Cultural Change

ALISON M.C. HENDERSON & JANICE M.A. MCMILLAN

Nottingham Trent University

AIMS

The focus of this paper is a study of several Health Authority and Health Board 'in-house' management, training and development programmes, which were provided between 1989 and 1991 to help develop managerial skills in healthcare staff. The aims of this paper are four-fold:

i. Firstly, we evaluate the contribution of 'in-house' management training programmes as a means of equipping healthcare staff with appropriate tools for operating in the new managerialist environment.

ii. Secondly we assess the impact of this type of management training and development on cultural change in the case-study organisations.

iii. Thirdly, we speculate on the implications for the further use of management training and development to help achieve long-lasting and deep-seated cultural change throughout the health service.

iv. Finally, we highlight issues pertinent to an agenda for further research into the mechanisms for achieving cultural change in the NHS.

INTRODUCTION

The UK National Health Service has undergone a lengthy series of fundamental organisational, structural and ideological changes during its forty-five year history. Arguably the most far-reaching and radical of these began in the 1980s with the injection of general management at all levels of the organisation, from Departmental

Managerial Issues in the Reformed NHS. Edited by M.Malek, P.Vacani, J.Rasquinha & P.Davey
© 1993 John Wiley & Sons Ltd

'Head Office' to front-line operations. The reforms impacted on English Health Authorities first in 1984; general managers were appointed in Scottish Health Boards in 1985. The changes received a major push with the so-called 'White-Paper' reforms in 1990. The introduction of internal markets, separating purchasers of healthcare from providers, and the creation of Trust status for provider units, and Fund-holding status for a selected and growing number of GP practices, were some of the more radical and significant structural, managerial, financial and ideological changes heralded by these reforms in both England and Scotland.

Such changes are acknowledged widely as major catalysts in the reform of NHS organisational culture, (Willcocks and Harrow, 1991; Lawton and Rose, 1991; Pollitt, 1989; Harrison, 1988; Klein, 1989; Strong and Robinson, 1988). There is a growing recognition that any organisational cultural change, including that which occurs in the NHS, is a lengthy, complex and convoluted process which needs to be managed from a variety of directions, and by a variety of methods, (Tietjen, 1991; Millar, 1991; Hassard and Sharifi, 1989; Richards, 1989; Deal and Kennedy, 1988;).

These issues suggest it is naive for any organisation's managers to rely on only one method. There is also a recognition that training should and can be utilised to achieve cultural change, (Deal and Kennedy, 1988; Pettigrew, 1990), although evaluations of the effectiveness of training, relative to other methods, have not been widely attempted. This will limit those same managers' judgement and understanding of the relative merits of cultural change strategies whilst encouraging them to focus on only one method. Furthermore, there is the assertion that it is easier to modify the manifestations of organisational culture, than it is to alter the core beliefs and assumptions which inform and shape them, but that any strategy for changing culture should aim to alter core beliefs as well as the more evident expressions of those beliefs, (Pettigrew, 1990; Richards, 1989). Such an assertion signals that cultural change strategies, to operate effectively, must induce change at both levels; and that strategies which do not operate in both levels may have limited effect. Of course, this assumes that it is possible to define the nature of, and differentiate between, the underlying beliefs and assumptions, and the resulting behavioural, structural and physical manifestations.

One of the key responses of the health service to the continued attempts to fashion a culture centred on an increasingly dominant ideology of managerialism, was to increase formal management training and development opportunities. Hence the need to focus on the impact of management training and development in achieving cultural change in the NHS.

Initially at least, the predominant emphasis in management development opportunities in English Health Authorities was on formal, and often short-term, in-house management training courses. In spite of earlier experiences which indicated the limitations of such an approach, Scottish Health Boards chose to respond to the introduction of general management by providing, in the main, similar formal management courses, and encouraging few other, if any, alternative cultural change strategies. In both the health boards studied, approximately ninety-five per cent of the management training provision was via in-house formalised training programmes.

This begs two questions. First of all, if Scottish Health Boards had known about, and taken on board, the experiences of their English colleagues, would they have put such emphasis on formal management courses of this type? Secondly, had they considered alternative means of developing staff to cope with the emerging managerial agenda, and if so, why did they focus on formal management training courses?

In addressing this research agenda, we draw on several sources: First, McMillan's, (1993), work on the impact of all the 'in-house' management training courses, at both board- and unit level, provided by two Scottish Health Boards during the period 1988 to 1991; these courses included two formal board-wide management training programmes which had been recently established, one in each board: The second source is the experiences of one of the authors who worked with two English Health Authorities on the learning needs of staff with managerial responsibilities, and the design and provision of management training and development opportunities which would help address those needs; these included 'in-house' short-term management skills training courses, an open learning version of the Open University course, "Managing Health Services", and a college-based postgraduate Diploma/M.BA (Health). The third source is information gleaned from the literature, including that which specifically addresses the issues of cultural change, and management training and development in the NHS.

ACHIEVING CULTURAL CHANGE

There is a growing literature which widens the debate on whether, and by what means, organisational culture can be managed, manipulated and changed. To understand the utility of management training to create cultural change, it is essential to define 'organisational culture'. At least two schools of thought can be identified. First, Schein (1975) views organisational culture as the underlying beliefs and assumptions, rather than their more obvious manifestations, such as behaviour, jargon, dress-codes. This contrasts with a wider definition of, for example, Wilson and Rosenfeld (1990) and Trice and Beyer (1984) which accepts these manifestations as part and parcel of organisational culture. In this paper, we work from the assumption that organisational culture is most readily conceptualised in layers: deeper stratifications of attitudes, beliefs and values which underpin the more superficial layers of behaviour, language, rituals, dress, decor, office layout, and workplace stories and legends. We also assume that the more deeply-seated layers of beliefs and values inform and fashion the nature of the more explicit and physical manifestations of culture.

Given the ability to define the nature of the elements of culture within the organisation, we should be able to identify how they alter over time, to indicate the depth of cultural change.

THE ROLE OF MANAGEMENT DEVELOPMENT AND TRAINING IN CULTURAL CHANGE

Achieving cultural change, may not appear to be one of the more frequently expressed aims of management training and development in organisations. More commonly expressed intentions focus on management development's contribution to ensuring that managers have adequate competences to meet present and future demands of their jobs. Armstrong (1991), among others, identifies several ways in which management development is said to increase the effectiveness of organisations. Rarely, is any explicit reference made to any potential that management development may have for altering or determining organisational culture; and when it is made, management development is considered to be only one of many mechanisms which can be deployed and which are deemed to be necessary, (Pettigrew, 1990).

DEFINING MANAGEMENT DEVELOPMENT AND TRAINING

For the purposes of this paper, we define management training as one vehicle of management development. We assume that management training can contribute to management development, but note that managers also learn and develop in other formal and informal ways, (Attwood *et al*, 1992; Margerison, 1991; Honey and Mumford, 1986; Pedler and Boydell, 1985; Mumford, 1971). We assume also that management development places a greater responsibility on individuals to self-learn, and is concerned with development of the whole person rather than merely the acquisition of a narrow set of defined skills and knowledge.

Often management development may be assumed to be synonymous with organisational development. Like management development and training, the definitions of organisational development can vary. Bennis (1969: 2) considers organisational development to be a "complex educational strategy intended to change the beliefs, attitudes, values and structures of organisations so they can better adapt to new technologies, new markets and challenges, and the dizzying rate of change itself." Yet, organisations are more than the sum of their managers.

Thus far, given the notion that management training represents only one of the formal vehicles of management development, and that management development is one strand only of an organisational development strategy, it follows that management training and development may have limited potential for achieving extensive *organisational* cultural change.

EVALUATING THE EFFECTIVENESS OF MANAGEMENT TRAINING AND DEVELOPMENT

The framework we use to investigate the effectiveness of management training courses comprises a simple model which defines the stages required for effective training. It has been adapted from an amalgam of Armstrong's generic models of systematic and planned training (Armstrong 1991), and from our experiences in designing and delivering management training and development programmes. The model is outlined in Table 1.

Table 1. Model to illustrate key stages for design and delivery of management training courses

Stage 1	Assess management development needs
Stage 2	Prioritise management development needs
Stage 3	Assess the type of management training and development required to address those needs
Stage 4	Select appropriately trained and experienced trainers to plan, design and implement training and development programmes
Stage 5	Evaluate management and training provided to ensure it is effective in meeting the desired impact

Adapted from Armstrong 1991: 421-422.

Although all the stages contribute to the overall effectiveness of any management training programme, stages 1 and 2 are crucial in driving those programmes in an appropriate direction. The direction should be indicated by the map of corporate goals and objectives.

Assessment of training needs can be determined at a number of levels including individual, role, department and organisation, and several approaches can be employed (Appelby 1991). It was thought that the training needs agenda, implied by contemporary organisational cultural reforms, required testing against the actual management training and development courses provided. It was also desired to examine the means by which training needs assessment was accomplished, and whether the identified needs addressed any particular level of culture at the expense of others.

EVALUATION OF MANAGEMENT TRAINING & DEVELOPMENT

"Everyone accepts the importance of evaluation in principle, but it is rarely carried out in practice" (Dearden 1986: 8). It would be extremely foolish to argue that evaluation is not the vital route to assessing whether the training and development has achieved the desired outcomes. What is less readily agreed, is the most effective way of evaluating training and development. Inevitably, it must be driven by the objectives set for the training and development experiences. All too often, evaluation of training and development centres on the 'feel good' factor, and an evaluation of the enjoyment of the delivery and gastronomic experiences (Maynard 1991).

The fault often lies with the choice of the level of evaluation, and many organisations tend to focus on evaluating the impact of training and development by testing participants' reactions rather than measure alterations in behaviour, practice, attitudes and values. Hamblin (1974) suggests five levels of evaluation; we use these to help construct a model to assess the evaluation methods used. Our model is illustrated in Table 2.

Table 2. Model to assess impact of methods used to evaluate Training and Development Courses

Provide information	Evaluation level	Process
Personal change at the individual level	1	document reactions of trainees
	2	measure what trainees have learned (knowledge/understanding)
	3	measure change in job behaviour of trainees (language/practice/skills/competences)
Organisational and Development	4	measure the effect the job Change behaviour changes at individual level have had on the functioning of the organisation
	5	measure ultimate value in terms of assessing the extent to which the organisation has benefited in achieving its success criteria

Adapted from Hamblin 1974:14

Hamblin suggests that the five levels represent stages in an overall process of evaluation, but that evaluation can start at any level. In terms of achieving cultural change, such a model has clear relevance. We suggest that the later stages provide information on the extent of organisational, as opposed to just personal, change and development. The earlier stages really focus on recording changes in the individual's language, work practices, knowledge and behaviour. Later stage evaluation thus provides valuable information which would illustrate the *depth* of the change in the elemental layers which comprise organisational culture.

The model is not intended to specify the means by which each stage can be achieved, as these will vary. Nor does it assess whether the desired outcomes of the training and development are known. Indeed, the crucial underlying assumption in any evaluation is that the organisation will use the results to compare against a known set of expected outcomes. The model does not specify a time-frame for evaluation. It is acknowledged that an activity such as management training and development may not always produce an immediate impact, (Dearden 1986). Furthermore, if the deeper-rooted aspects of cultural change take longer to achieve, we assert that it is important for organisations to aim for longer-term evaluation, particularly in levels 4 and 5, as well.

BACKGROUND INFORMATION ON STUDY ORGANISATIONS

Two Scottish and two English health authorities were studied. One Scottish health board served a population of approximately 500,000 and employed almost 13,000 staff, and the other, a population of approximately 345,000 with a staff of some 7500 employees. One of the English health authorities served a population of just over 600,000 with a staff of approximately 15,000, and the other, a population of almost 285,000 with a staff of 4,500.

FINDINGS
Training Needs Assessment

There was a marked distinction between the Scottish and English authorities in relation to the extent of training needs assessment. In both Scottish health boards, there was no apparent evidence of any systematic and comprehensive training needs assessment.

In the case of one Scottish health board, the missed opportunity arose when the Board embarked on a major information-gathering exercise in 1986, which was planned as the first stage in the establishment of an organisation development (OD) programme. From a survey of around 1000 staff, 16 key managerial issues such as communication, training and strategy, were identified (Fullerton and Price, 1991). These highlighted the problems of some 1,000 staff from all levels of the organisation. The OD programme was geared to introduce and/or improve procedures and systems to counteract problems in the internal organisation environment. Whilst training as an issue was highlighted, it was subsequently tackled in isolation from the other issues raised by the survey. Consequently, attempts to define a training programme were constrained by this lack of integration with the remaining key managerial issues on the OD programme. Furthermore, subsequent training topics were neither prioritised nor analysed in terms of the management training and the development needs of staff at different levels of the organisation.

In the other Scottish board, the management training needs assessment appears to have been a cerebral exercise carried out by the senior management team of the health board. The content of management training programmes carried out at board- wide level was strongly driven by the training course tenders proffered by various training providers. At no point was there an explicit statement of management training needs. The management training programme tenders were selected on the basis of perceived value-for-money. This measure was a marker set by those senior managers involved in the award of the tender with no reference to any current, management training needs perceived by staff. In this case, the 'better' tender (in terms of relevance of training) was passed over in favour of a cheaper alternative. It is possible that the decision to opt for a cheaper tender was based not on organisationally-imposed cash limits, but rather on the notion that the organisation was not certain of the full extent of its management training needs, so could not reasonably evaluate the added value, if any, from a more expensive tender. The fact that the cheapest tender was not rejected on grounds of cost, but on inadequate content, at least indicates a limited acknowledgement of the relevance of training needs assessment.

With reference to our first model, the linear progression may well have broken down in the early stages in the Scottish boards: Even when stages 1 and 2 are carried out to a limited extent, we can challenge the effectiveness of the methods used by the organisation. If stages 1 and 2 determine the effectiveness of subsequent stages, we can already predict the limited success of the programmes in achieving cultural change.

The English authorities provided a different perspective. District and unit-wide surveys of perceived management training needs comprised one of the first steps to achieve cultural change. This process often resulted in an extensive list of generic management training needs, (often up to 40 in number), which were then refined to match the needs of staff at different levels. There were systematic attempts to identify management development and training requirements in terms of both organisational and individual needs. The mechanisms of surveys, staff appraisal and individual performance review provided channels through which individual training needs assessment were identified. In one unit, this was piloted by focusing on two specific staff groups, Ward Managers and Deputy Ward Managers. The pilot survey resulted in the identification of ten key sets of organisational needs, (including HRM, Financial Management, Impact of New Legislation, Ethics in Health Care and Total Quality Management), and six key sets of individual needs, (including time management, problem solving, decision making, team building and inter agency working), Representative Ward and Deputy Ward Managers then worked with line managers, training managers and trainers to refine and prioritise those needs and construct tailored training packages. With reference to our first model, the linear progression was strengthened by the explicit recognition of both authorities of the importance of stages 1 and 2, and the efforts made to execute them effectively.

Meeting Management Training Needs

In one Scottish board, it was expected that all managers down to supervisor level would receive a minimum of fifteen hours management training per year via either the board-wide programme or alternative internal and external courses. The board-wide programme offered four identical phases, each of four days of training in performance appraisal only, and was not stated to be compulsory. However, managers were strongly recommended to undertake the course, and a total of 400 attended the first two phases. In the other Scottish board, the board-wide management training programme was compulsory for an identified group of 600 managers. The programme ran over two-and-a-half years, and each manager undertook three one-week modules. During that time, the uptake of other in-house management training courses was severely curtailed.

In the absence of a clear identification of management training needs in the Scottish authorities, it was necessary to construct a framework to examine the appropriateness of the management training provided. McMillan (1993), examined the skills required by public sector managers in response to central government legislative changes and initiatives since 1979, and the consequent internal organisational changes in the health boards. Seven key management training areas for managers were identified:

- financial management,
- value for money (VFM),
- communication,
- human resources management (HRM),
- planning, evaluation and compulsory competitive tendering for ancillary services (CCT).

For each board these training areas were further refined to define the precise training needs under each of these seven headings.

The content of all in-house management training courses offered was examined and compared against the training needs analyses described above. This analysis revealed no incidence of in-house training provision in evaluation and CCT in the Scottish boards studied. This was clearly linked to the failure to identify these as training needs. And, the emphasis of one board-wide programme on training managers to carry out performance appraisal further constrained the ability of the authority to meet the fuller range of training needs.

In the English authorities, there were clear attempts to allow the outcomes of the training needs assessment processes to drive the content of the subsequent array of management development and training programmes. Furthermore, although both authorities provided distance and open learning management development programmes centred on the Open University course, "Managing Health Services", they supplemented these considerably with a range of short-term formal in-house management training courses at both district and unit level, as well as other courses designed and run by external providers. In one authority, a Postgraduate Diploma/M.BA (Health) programme was established in conjunction with the health authority. Two cohorts, each of sixteen students, have so far been recruited to that part-time, but intensive, management education and development programme.

Evaluation of the Management Training and Development Programmes

The most striking overall finding was the limited post-course evaluation of each of the management training and development programmes. It consisted, in the main, of immediate post-event feedback from the trainees via what the authors have termed 'happy sheets'. These recorded the trainees immediate impressions of relevance, delivery styles, location of training and general facilities.

In the Scottish boards, this written feedback was frequently left unanalysed and was retained by the trainers themselves. One further mechanism of pre-course briefing and post-course debriefing was used in the Scottish boards. In one, these sessions consisted of face to face interviews between the participants and their immediate line supervisors. However, there were no means of assessing change in behaviour over a longer post-course period. Furthermore, there was no formal expectation that information gleaned from these sessions would be transmitted back to those with responsibilities for management training provision. In the majority of cases, no information was sent back. In the other board, not all courses were subject even to this feedback mechanism, and, when it did occur, there was no evidence of mechanisms which would have ensured the use and analysis of this information to improve further training. With reference to our second model, it was evident that much, if not all, of the documented evaluation was restricted to level 1 in the Scottish boards studied.

In the English authorities, there were some attempts to survey the perceived changes in managerial practice some six months after completion of a course. However, this exercise was never evaluated, nor the comments disseminated to staff in the organisation. With reference to our second model, most evaluation is restricted to level 1. In some of the courses, the existence of formal assessment by examination allows a partial evaluation characteristic level 2. It should be noted that the formal staff appraisal process allowed informal evaluation more akin to level 3 to occur. This information was not necessarily fed back to those with responsibility for designing and delivering the management training and development programmes.

IMPLICATIONS

Whatever the ultimate contribution of management training and development to organisational cultural change, the effectiveness of the in-house management training and development courses studied is constrained by several factors.

The first of these constraints is the failure to assess training needs and the use of inadequate methods. The overall approach suggests that a collation of individually perceived impressions of need, however random and unique, can readily become assumed to be the framework for the organisation's management development programme. Often missing is a diagnosis of the skills, competences, behaviour and attitudes required to function effectively in a desired future organisational culture. This would require an identifiable relationship to be made between the priorities set by the organisation's corporate goals and individually perceived training needs. Certainly, the potential contribution that management training and development makes to changing organisational culture will be partly driven by the extent to which this 'fit' is made. All too often organisations fall into the trap of isolating the identification of training needs from overall corporate goals, and the gap between present and desired cultures. Furthermore, the seductiveness of the process of training needs analysis needs to be recognised; it can often become a surrogate for the process of identifying the elements of the desired organisational culture and goals. The training and development programmes become viewed as an end of cultural change rather than a means of achieving it.

The second constraint is the relevance of the training provided in terms of skills and competences targeted. The danger is that, in the absence of a systematic and comprehensive training needs assessment, the likelihood of identifying inappropriate priorities, increases. As one example, the current NHS cultural reforms have far-reaching consequences for the extent to which clinicians, (notably consultants and GPs), must adopt managerial roles. Yet, even in the organisations studied, the targeting of clinicians for the management training courses studied was lower than might have reasonably been expected given that the success of the cultural reforms will be partly determined by the extent to which medical sub-cultures shift towards and adopt the emergent managerialist paradigm.

The third constraint is the level of post-course evaluation. The ability to evaluate the effectiveness and impact of the management training and development courses in the organisations studied has been severely constrained by the nature of the evaluation carried out. Evaluation, designed to establish immediate reactions and type of knowledge gained, restricts the information available with which to measure the extent of changes in working practices, behaviours, attitudes and values. Furthermore, training and development may be driving the cultural changes, yet it is hard to envisage how the present evaluation methods can hope to conclusively demonstrate this one way or the other.

CONCLUSIONS AND ISSUES FOR A RESEARCH FRAMEWORK

Our work prompts several key issues about the extent to which management training and development can be used to help achieve cultural change in health organisations. These are pertinent to our framework for future research.

Firstly, if we accept the layered composition of organisational culture, we can question the extent to which the vehicle of training courses impact on each layer. In particular, can training bring about and sustain the deep-seated modifications in values, beliefs and attitudes of staff ? Some claim that language is a key medium through which culture is transmitted in an organisation, (Pettigrew, 1990). Training and development courses do provide one means through which staff can be exposed to new ideas via a new language; following training, some staff may even adopt and start to promulgate the 'new' language. The question is whether other mechanisms are required to re-inforce and sustain these changes until such a time when the deeper-rooted and longer-term changes in beliefs and attitudes occur.

Secondly, the impact of training may be linked to the Hawthorne effect - it may not just be the training itself which induces change; those receiving training and development can feel more valued and open to new concepts and the development of new skills. However, the risk is that training and development raises issues which run counter to the existing organisational culture, or the 'spin' of the organisation, (Fairbairns, 1991:44). The consequence is that, on return to work, the new ideas, skills and behaviours may be undermined, challenged and lost. Unless reinforced by other staff and organisation systems, staff exposed to the training may rapidly lose heart, become cynical and consider it a waste of effort to change. In other words, management training and development courses may enable the organisation to signal explicitly a change in culture, and initiate the change process. But there is a danger that the management training and development courses can become the panacea for handling learning and development associated with achieving change in the organisation. The question arises as to the most effective ways of reinforcing the change induced by training and development courses. There is a growing recognition that other mechanisms such as action learning, managerial leadership and innovation management may sustain the continued learning process among work-based teams. Further work is required to evaluate the relative contributions of these other organisational cultural change agents and mechanisms in supplementing training and development courses in the achievement of organisational cultural change.

A third issue emerges from the specific question as to how effective management training and development are in dismantling the cultural barriers between the professional tribes which are still a feature of today's NHS. The instance of one English authority which targeted peer groups of staff from horizontal layers within individual professional hierarchies, highlights the potential risk of reinforcing existing, and creating new tribes. After initial training and development in the peer group, this risk might be reduced by facilitating joint learning and application in actual work-based teams which cut across professional and hierarchical boundaries. The impact of this needs to be further evaluated.

And finally, a fourth issue centres on the impact that management training and development can make in inculcating a managerialist culture among staff from clinical professions. Does management training and development need to a precursor to clinical training? The nature of current clinical professional training tends to establish and re-inforce tribal boundaries; managerial issues, skills and competences in health are more generic in nature than those of individual clinical professions, and require inter-disciplinary understanding and learning. It may well be easier to address these before the characteristic and distinctive professional cultures have been established.

It is unlikely that the creation of a true learning organisation is achieved by the sole means of training and development programmes. Nonetheless, management training and development could be valuable vehicles which help contribute to effective cultural change in health organisations, so long as the trap of isolating these means from other vehicles of organisational cultural change is avoided.

REFERENCES

Appelby, R. C. (1991), Modern Business Administration, Pitman, London.

Armstrong, M. (1991), A Handbook of Personnel Management, Kogan Page Publishing, London.

Attwood, M., Hewitt, I., and Key, P. (1992), 'The Loneliness of the Long-Distance Manager', Health Services Management, November/December 1992, 21-23.

Bennis, W. G. (1969), Organization and Development: its nature, origins and prospects, Addison-Wesley Publishing Company, USA.

Deal, T. and Kennedy, A. A. (1988), Corporate Cultures: The Rites and Rituals of Corporate Life, Penguin Books.

Dearden, R. (1986), 'Standard recognition', The Health Service Journal, 27 November 1986, 7-8.

Fairbairns, J. (1991), 'Plugging the Gap in Training Needs Analysis' Personnel Management, February 1991, 43-45.

Fullerton, H. and Price, C. (1991), 'Culture Change in the NHS', Personnel Management, March 1991, 50-53.

Hamblin, A. C. (1991), Evaluation and Control of Training, McGraw-Hill, London.

Harrison, S. (1988), Managing the National Health Service, Chapman Hall, London.

Hassard, J. and Sharifi, S. (1989), 'Corporate Culture and Strategic Change', Journal of General Management, 15/2, 4-19.

Honey, P. and Mumford A. (1986), A Manual of Learning Styles, Honey, London.

Klein, R. (1989), The Politics of the NHS, Longman, London and New York.

Lawton, A. and Rose, A. (1991), Organisation and Management in the Public Sector, Pitman Publishing, London.

McMillan, J. M. A. (1993), 'Improving Public Sector Management Training in Scotland', PhD thesis, Robert Gordon University, Aberdeen, for submission October 1993.

Margerison, C. (1991), Making Management Development Work, The McGraw-Hill Training Series, London.

Mark, A. and Scott, H. (1991), 'Management in the National Health Service', Willcocks, L. and Harrow, J. (eds), Rediscovering Public Service Management, McGraw-Hill, Maidenhead, England, 197-234.

Maynard, A. (1991), 'Making a monkey of us', Health Service Journal, 26 September 1991, 21.

Millar, B. (1991), 'Knowledge by Degrees', The Health Service Journal, 4 April 1991, 23-25.

Mumford, A. (1971), The Manager and Training, Pitman, London.

Pedler, M. and Boydell, T. (1985), Managing Yourself, Fontana, London.

Pettigrew, A. M. (1990), 'Is Corporate Culture Manageable?', Wilson, C. and Rosenfeld, R. (eds), Managing Organisations: Texts, Readings and Cases, McGraw-Hill, Berkshire, England, 266-272.

Pollitt, C. (1989), 'New Wave Public Service Reforms', The Health Service Journal, 27 April 1989, 3-4.

Richards, S. (1989), 'The Course of Cultural Change', The Health Service Journal, 27 April 1989, 1-2.

Schein, E. H. (1985), Organisational Culture and Leadership, Jossey-Bass, San Francisco.

Strong, P. and Robinson, J. (1990), The NHS under New Management, Open University Press, Buckingham, England.

Tietjen, C. (1991), 'Management Development in the NHS', Personnel Management, May 1991, 2-5.

Trice, H. M. and Beyer, J. M. (1984), 'Studying Organisational Cultures Through Rites and Ceremonials', Academy of Management Review, 9, 653-669.

15 A Monitoring and Evaluation Framework for the Implementation of 'The Health of the Nation'

GEOFF H.D. ROYSTON

Economics and Operational Research Division, Department of Health

The Health of the Nation set out a strategy for health in England. The White Paper gave a commitment to monitoring and reviewing progress with the strategy and outlined how this would be done. Some of the promised actions are already well underway. This paper develops that outline and sets those actions into a fuller monitoring and evaluation framework.

The Government's overall goal in Health of the Nation is to secure continuing improvement in the general health of the population in England by adding years to life and adding life to years. It envisages success through:

1. Public policies that consider the health dimension, by the active promotion of healthy surroundings
2. By increasing knowledge and understanding of healthy lifestyles (and enabling people to act upon this)
3. By the provision of high quality health services based on identified health needs
4. An appropriate balance between health promotion, disease prevention, treatment, care, and rehabilitation.

These general goals have been operationalised by selecting five key areas:

*   Coronary heart disease/stroke;
*   Cancers;
*   Mental illness;
*   HIV/AIDS and sexual health;
*   Accidents.

These were where there was believed to be the greatest need and scope for cost-effective improvement in over all health, and, by setting for these priority areas

Managerial Issues in the Reformed NHS. Edited by M.Malek, P.Vacani, J.Rasquinha & P.Davey
© 1993 John Wiley & Sons Ltd

specific, generally quantitative, mortality, morbidity and risk factor targets to be met by given dates. These goals, priorities and, especially, targets provide a clear focus for monitoring and evaluation work. The primary question must be: *are things on track for achieving the targets?* This paper sets out a framework for addressing that question. Throughout this paper the terms monitoring and evaluation have frequently been used together. In principle monitoring is more to do with checking progress on implementation, and evaluation with assessing its results, but the two are inevitably linked.

AIMS AND COVERAGE OF MONITORING AND EVALUATION

The purpose of monitoring and evaluative work is to provide assurance that the necessary implementation steps are being taken, to establish that the desired outcomes are being achieved, and to enable any necessary improvements. A secondary aim might be to disentangle the effects of Health of the Nation from other initiatives — Working for Patients, Promoting Better Health, etc. There may be limited aspects where some evaluative steps in this direction would be feasible, for example, in comparing progress on targets against previous trends or predictions of future trends, or in considering specific Health of the Nation initiatives. However, rigorous and comprehensive evaluation of this sort would be an impossible task. Even if it were not so, it would probably be a misguided one. Working for Patients for example, provides a platform for Health of the Nation. As the White Paper points out, some health outcomes will take time to emerge clearly. It will therefore be important to monitor progress on the development of the structures and processes which help generate the improvements in health. Elaborating on a Health of the Nation context yields a monitoring and evaluation chain (actually an iterative loop), the main links of which are:

- Enabling actions (infrastructure) needed to support interventions
- Direct interventions at population or individual level
- Intermediate outcomes of interventions, such as behavioural change
- Disease (or accident) outcomes such as precursors or incidence of illness
- Main health target outcomes, mainly mortality

The primary indicators of the success of the Health of the Nation are the outcome targets for the key areas. Most of these are mortality targets, but some relate to changes in disease levels, in peoples' behaviour or in other risk factors. The mixed nature of the Health of the Nation targets, together with the time taken for health outcomes (such as the change in mortality) change to emerge clearly, demonstrates that the four *progress* (or supplementary) links of the monitoring and evaluation chain will have as vital a role as the final health outcome link (Work on such indicators is underway). Inclusion of progress aspects (which, as shown above, includes not only structural and process but also some outcome elements) of monitoring and evaluation is not just a practical necessity, it should allow a deeper understanding of what is driving progress towards targets and therefore of identifying examples of good practice and what needs to be done where progress is unsatisfactory.

A realistic and useful set of objectives for monitoring and evaluation of Health of the Nation therefore would be to allow the Department to assess:

- Whether the process is on track to meet the main health outcome targets, as measured (mainly) by changes in mortality
- Whether the necessary changes are taking place in related disease incidence or precursors
- Whether the process is on track to meet the behavioural and other non-clinical risk factor targets, and to achieve any other changes required in such areas but not explicitly set as targets
- What direct interventions, authorities and others are making at population or individual level in pursuit of Health of the Nation goals and targets
- How well authorities are progressing with enabling action or infrastructure building to support such interventions
- What ,and why, any problems were occurring, and, by identifying good practice or otherwise, how they might be surmounted

The main areas set out in the White Paper where monitoring and evaluation are necessary are:

(a) *The key areas*; coronary heart disease, mental illness, and so on.
(b) *Cross-cutting work (mostly) outside the NHS;* healthy alliances, healthy settings, guidance on policy appraisal and health, professional education and training etc.
(c) *Other work within or for the NHS;* central support for local development (e.g. focus groups, handbooks), local target setting, health education, healthy hospitals, NHS R&D etc.

In principle, questions on health outcomes, risk factor (disease and intermediate) outcomes, direct interventions, and, infrastructure can be asked in any area. In practice, health outcome and risk factor questions are likely to predominate in the key areas, and intervention and infrastructure ones on the cross-cutting work. The following sections of this paper discuss the above three areas in turn. Note that the examples given are illustrative and partial, *not* comprehensive. The discussion necessarily covers a lot of ground in a short space; separate monitoring and evaluation protocols may be needed in many of these areas.

KEY AREAS

Assessing progress towards *health outcome* targets in the key areas is the fundamental monitoring and evaluation issue. For each target such as: 'reducing death rates in both CHD and stroke in people under 65 by at least 40% by the year

2000', national progress will need to be tracked. Work on such monitoring and evaluation of outcomes in the key areas is well underway. An example is the publication of the Specification of National Indicators and the extension to the Public Health Common Basic Dataset. However, as already mentioned *risk factor—intermediate and disease outcome* indicators will be needed. Some of these will be leading indicators of which the question will need to be asked: 'does their rate of movement point to achievement of the primary targets?' As suggested above, the Health of the Nation risk factor targets, e.g.: 'reducing the prevalence of cigarette smoking to no more than 20% by the year 2000 in both men and women', might be considered as progress or supplementary indicators. But there will be many others to be developed and monitored such as. the distribution of blood pressure on GPs lists, or the reduction in major strokes in those with transient ischaemic attack.

Although risk factors and health outcomes are the focus here, it may well be appropriate also to assess the reaction of the public, employers, and the institutions to the associated interventions. As part of any cost-effectiveness estimation work, it may also be possible to assess value for money aspects of Health of the Nation initiatives. As well as monitoring and evaluation of health and risk factor outcomes, the *direct interventions* for populations or individuals that are taken to produce these outcomes in the key areas will need to be assessed. (These would include health promotion and preventative intervention by alliances, by work in 'healthy settings', and by NHS professionals). To complement more detailed tracking of such activity, general monitoring will be needed of the shifts of the balance of resources from secondary treatment to primary prevention.

It would, probably not be appropriate to include research into the effectiveness of particular interventions as part of monitoring and evaluating Health of the Nation (such work is of course vital, but forms part of a larger canvas). Monitoring of interventions has to be more *downstream* and will involve such questions as: 'are interventions that are known to be effective being used?, or 'are they reaching the relevant individuals or populations?. Examples would include, the percentage of smokers on GPs lists who are receiving advice on smoking, the proportion of patients who have had heart attacks that are receiving follow-up aspirin therapy, or the onset-to-needle time in acute heart attacks. Some of the *enabling actions*; such as building infrastructure needed to support interventions in Key Areas will be built as a result of cross-cutting work. But there will be some more specific Key Area related aspects, particularly:

- Training staff
- Integrating health gain objectives into contracting mechanisms
- Aligning GP contracts to key area objectives
- Developing information and information systems
- Development of good practice protocols and guidelines

The main generic monitoring and evaluation questions on infrastructure should address if the piece of infrastructure has been built, and if the desired activity is flowing from it.

Infrastructure monitoring and evaluation that is particularly relevant to key areas might include such questions as: what percentage of emergency ambulances are crewed by paramedics?, what percentage of the workforce are covered by no-smoking in the workplace policies?, Has the health authority carried out a lifestyle survey?, and, is there a local stroke or heart attack register?

CROSS-CUTTING WORK (MOSTLY) OUTSIDE THE NHS

As well as monitoring and evaluation work *within* the Key Areas, there will need to be an assessment of progress *across* them. Health of the Nation extends beyond the traditional health context, as for example into many aspects of employment and industry. The White Paper set out a number of key actors among whom joint action and healthy alliances would be promoted. Outside the NHS, these actors included:

- Government
- Local Authorities
- The Health Education Authority
- The Confederation of British Industry
- The Trades Union Congress
- The Research Community
- Voluntary Organisations
- The Media

Additionally the White Paper noted the opportunities for pursuing action in the places where people live and work as healthy settings. Outside the NHS these include cities, schools, workplaces, homes, and prisons,

The White Paper noted also the variations in health in particular groups of people within the population and the need to consider their particular needs and concerns. Such groups were:

- Infants and children
- Elderly people
- Women
- Black and ethnic minority groups
- Socio-economic groups
- People with physical, sensory or learning disabilities
- Other groups e.g. carers or homeless people

Cross-cutting work includes some of the Departmental White Paper commitments such as promoting healthy alliances, reviewing the strategic aims of the Health Education Authority, examining ways of supporting the UK Healthy Cities network, developing professional education and training on disease prevention and health promotion, and building international links on health strategy

Full monitoring and evaluation of the work of *healthy alliances* and in *healthy settings* will be a major challenge, requiring the development of novel instruments and indicators and raising difficult issues of accountability. It is for example unlikely that many useful *quantitative* indicators will be found here. A more realistic aim might be to ensure that indicators of progress are *specific*. Monitoring and evaluation of the early stages of cross-cutting work should be relatively straightforward, as the main generic questions are the same as mentioned in the previous section (Has this piece of infrastructure been built? Is the desired activity flowing from it?) Examples might include:

- Has a pilot network of health promoting schools been developed?
- Have they produced and shared strategies for changing pupils' behaviour?
- Are these strategies being implemented?, or, more local examples might be: have local and health authorities formed a joint heart health strategy?, and are they funding joint local projects to progress it?

THE NHS

The unique position of the NHS in promoting health was of course recognised in the White Paper. The NHS will be expected to establish a more direct link between what it does and results in terms of individual and population health. The White Paper outlined required action to this end at various levels, ranging from the community provider units, and primary and community health care services.

Particular NHS actions cited in the White Paper which will need monitoring and evaluation include work on *healthy hospitals*, NHS research and development, and setting of local priorities and targets

The last of these three items has a particular importance for evaluation and monitoring. There is a strong connection between local health priorities and targets and indeed, national monitoring and evaluation. The former provides a key focus for the latter. But the points made about the need for progress indicators apply even more strongly at local level, where time horizons may be shorter and 'small numbers' problems larger in magnitude. Key monitoring and evaluation questions on local targets will include

- Are local targets compatible with national targets?
- Are they achievable in the light of local conditions and opportunities?
- Do they present any perverse incentives?
- Can accountability be reasonably ascribed?
- Is the required health outcome and progress information available?

Local target setting is a major topic in its own right and a discussion paper on it is being prepared.

As well as monitoring and evaluation of NHS activity, the role of the NHS in monitoring and evaluation itself needs to be considered. Monitoring and evaluation of Health of the Nation has vital local aspects, at regional, district, hospital and community levels. There will need to be, as for all NHS performance monitoring, a tiered approach which avoids inappropriately detailed oversight from the centre i.e.: the NHS Management Executive monitors performance of regions, regions monitor DHAs and FHSAs, DHAs and FHSAs monitor their own progress. Much of this framework will have some relevance to monitoring and evaluation at those levels. Progress on the actions outlined in the White Paper for each level will need to be monitored. Different indicators and instruments may be appropriate at each level, while keeping the number of indicators manageable, and the scale of monitoring and evaluation activity in proportion to the scale of the activity itself will be imported. Information will need to flow between different levels. The NHSME "DISP" project is addressing information requirements and information flows. The products of some initial work on implementation of Health of the Nation in the NHS are already in existence. The NHSME has recently published a report (First Steps for the NHS) on the work of the Health of the Nation *Focus Groups*, setting out possible local actions which the NHS might take, through regional, district and FHSA contracts, and through provider business plans, in each Key Area. Regions have produced initial Health of the Nation implementation plans. Detailed handbooks on each of the Key Areas have just been published.

A number of lessons for monitoring and evaluation for the NHS are emerging from this work. There is a general need to stimulate monitoring, audit and evaluation, focused on the Key Areas, at all levels of the service and to arrange feedback achievements against Health of the Nation objectives. This feedback is crucial both to improve the quality of the information as well as to support monitoring and evaluation as an iterative process. Regular review mechanisms will need to be established. Corporate contracts and purchasing plans will be an essential tool for annual (or more frequent) monitoring. Local objectives, as well as consequent management tasks and timetables will need to be set and criteria for assessing their achievement established. Other points that need to be observed are:

(a) Ensuring that contracts at RHA, DHA, and FHSA levels, together with purchasing negotiations, NHS contracts and provider business plans, give systematic coverage of monitoring and evaluation arrangements

(b) The need to improve information systems to enable baselines to be established, targets to be set, and progress monitored, especially for risk factors for which there are no routine information systems at local level

(c) The need to improve ability to monitor the effectiveness and cost-effectiveness of interventions, including intermediate measures of progress, and to develop proxy measures of health improvement

(d) The consideration of the need for lifestyle surveys to support monitoring and policy development

(e) The identification and dissemination of examples of good practice, including the role of annual Public Health Reports in this process

(f) Identifying marker issues against which progress could be measured

(g) Links to Health Authority information strategies and the development of Health of the Nation information strategy

(h) Joint involvement of health and social services in monitoring

(i) The participation of patients in (for example) functional health status assessment

(j) The involvement of groups independent of health or social services in monitoring, particularly organisations reporting to or run by users

TROUBLESHOOTING

The above monitoring and evaluation will produce a variety of information and insights which should make it easier for problems to be overcome. But this could be considerably enhanced by a systematic and comprehensive approach to garnering examples of good practice and to then disseminating them in a usable way. This would be a very natural and straightforward extension of what has been outlined so far. It also adds in the key questions: what problems are there, and why are they happening?, and what are examples of good practice?. Mechanisms for such garnering and dissemination will need to be established.

WIDER ISSUES

There is a case for including some rather wider issues in the evaluation of the implementation of Health of the Nation. Such wider questions might refer back to the overall goals (years to life and life to years) and the steps to them cited in the introduction. In addition a wider look could include questions such as, what are the costs of achievement?, are there any adverse side-effects (including opportunity costs) or beneficial spin-offs?, are any amendments to goals, objectives, priorities or targets indicated?, and, has the process of priority and target setting proved useful? There are also likely to be monitoring and evaluation questions about inter-relations within or between key areas, cross-cutting, and NHS aspects. For monitoring, this points to the need to establish an implementation 'project network' or 'map' to help with the co-ordination, scheduling and resourcing of the various activities. For evaluation, it points to the need for analytical and modelling work to help look at the interactions between targets.

Experience in the World Health Organisation has been that evaluation gives a clearer picture when compared with experience in other countries, especially in the field of alliance building and 'healthy settings'. Consideration is being given to the place of such comparative work for Health of the Nation.

SUPPORTING METHODS AND INFORMATION

The White Paper stated the Government's intention to publish a detailed appraisal of information and indicators needed to monitor progress in each Key Area. It gave commitments to a number of other actions to assist monitoring and evaluation including

- Expanded national health surveys
- A NHS survey advisory centre
- A new series of epidemiological overviews by the CHMU
- Development of a Public Health Information Strategy
- The enhancement of Directors of Public Health annual health reports to help monitor, review and develop the strategy for health
- Development of health outcome indicators and the Outcomes Clearing House
- Orientation of research towards health strategy aims
  (Progress on these actions is itself a candidate for monitoring and evaluation!)

Common tasks for such initiatives will be:
- To establish what information is required for monitoring and evaluating Health of the Nation
- To ascertain what relevant information is available from what sources, and to collate, analyse and disseminate it
- To identify the major gaps in required information; including its coverage, consistency and comparability
- To show how those gaps might most efficiently and cost-effectively be filled
- To help fill them, or demonstrate how to manage without filling them

The main issues about methods and information are likely to concern:
- Indicators e.g. primary health outcome and supplementary progress measures
- Dimensions e.g. client group, intervention type
- Instruments e.g. routine data, surveys

REPORTING ARRANGEMENTS

The White Paper commitment to 'periodic reports' and 'regular reviews' will need to be firmed up to indicate

- Frequency and timing
- Content
- Dissemination/audience

One possibility would be for the periodic reports to concentrate on monitoring matters, and the reviews to focus on evaluation. Whatever is decided it will be important to ensure that results are be presented in a way that facilitates their application to decision making![1]

---

[1] The contents of this paper express the author's view alone and in no way commit the Department of Health

16 Contracting, Planning, Competition and Efficiency

JOSEP FIGUERAS, JENNIFER A. ROBERTS, COLIN F. SANDERSON

London School of Hygiene and Tropical Medicine

INTRODUCTION

Contracting has been defined as *"a mutual agreement between two or more parties that something shall be done or forborne by one or both"* (Oxford English Dictionary, 1933). Where the matter at issue is a service, a contract is a formal written agreement which sets out conditions on what the provider is to supply, and on what and how the purchaser will pay for it (DoH, 1989). Evidently this requires organisational separation between those setting the conditions and paying, and those agreeing to the conditions and being paid.

The use of contracting in the health care sector is not new. For many years it has been the main method of funding services provided through, for example, private insurance companies in the US and the sickness funds in Germany. Yet the introduction of provider or internal markets within health care systems that have explicit social objectives such as equity and meeting needs, both in the British NHS (DoH, 1990) and in other several European countries (Wynand, 1989; CAE, 1991; Saltman, 1992) has given contracting a new dimension.

Contracting constitutes the central element of the new NHS organizational structure, regulating the relationship between purchasers and providers. It is based on the somewhat naive paradigm that market forces will invariably lead to improvements in efficiency and quality of services (Culyer, 1990). The argument put forward here is that the real impact of contracting lies in its potential as an instrument for translating plan objectives into real changes in the provision of care and funding them accordingly.

PLANNING'S ACHILLES' HEEL

From its beginnings in 1976 (DHSS, 1976a), there have been gaps in the NHS planning system. Even where priorities, plans and programmes have been worked

Managerial Issues in the Reformed NHS. Edited by M.Malek, P.Vacani, J.Rasquinha & P.Davey
© 1993 John Wiley & Sons Ltd

out, change in the real world has been slow, absent, or even perverse. The main reason for this has been an inadequate set of mechanisms for translating plans into action in the face of resistance from health care providers. Planning has tended to have been separated from the financing and management functions, and to have had little influence on them. The weakness of the link with financing in particular has been described as *"the Achilles' heel of contemporary planning practice"* (Rodwin, 1984).

The introduction of programme budgeting (PB) by the Department of Health aimed to establish an explicit link between planning and financing (DHSS, 1976b; DHSS 1977). PB had three ends in view: first, to improve planning decisions, through better assessments of financial implications of the options being considered; second, to establish guidelines on resource allocation according to the objectives and priorities; and third, to monitor and control the implementation of objectives and priorities. However PB failed to meet its objectives. At present, while not officially abandoned, its only legacy is a set of `care group' headings used for reporting and accounting purposes.

PB faced two major methodological problems. First, the classification of programmes adopted - based on client and service groups - meant that some programmes served several client groups, e.g. Primary Health Care (Jones, 1987). Moreover, it was argued that the size of some programmes e.g. acute and general services programme was too large to be meaningful (Glennerster, 1983). Second, there were methodological problems measuring costs, activities and benefits and assigning them to programmes which resulted in a lack of confidence in the information produced by PB.

More importantly, it could be argued that even if the methodological problems were solved, PB would still fail to achieve its objectives. The centralist and rational nature of PB exacerbates the organizational problems generating conflict and resistance to change. The latter is illustrated by the resistance of clinicians to the first DHSS guidelines on PB (Rathwell, 1987).

CONTRACTING AND ORGANIZATIONAL CHANGES IN THE NHS

The organizational changes that came with the introduction of contracting in the British NHS have had an important impact on the scope of decision-making at different levels with the hierarchy.

Decisions relating to technical or production efficiency have been shifted towards managers within provider organizations; the activities of the old health authorities in this field, as expressed in their `efficiency programmes' are in decline, particularly as the numbers of hospitals becoming independent trusts has increased. This shift can be seen as an extension of the thinking behind the introduction of general management following the Griffiths reforms (DHSS, 1983), but with new scope for introducing internal change and incentives and, in theory at least, the added stimulus of competition.

The knowledge and authority of clinicians, and the dangers of treating them as objects to be planned around has been recognised in the move to draw them into both management and tendering processes. Under the resource management initiative (Packwood, 1991) they are treated as the 'natural managers' of the NHS, with new organizational structures and information systems to facilitate their participation. Clinicians also need to agree to the financial and workload implications of the contracts covering their fields, and in some hospitals clinical directorates are directly involved in the contracting process as the ultimate provider to ensure that *"in an attempt to win contracts managers do not offer more than clinicians can - or want to -achieve"* (Roberts, 1993). The risk is that this may result in organisational fragmentation, new forms of tribalism and a lack of cooperation between clinical directorates (Rea, 1992).

At the same time, important aspects of decisions relating to the balance of 'goods' produced have been shifted away from clinicians and towards the new purchasing organisations, with their responsibilities for `assessments of need'. Contracts are the instrument for making providers increasingly accountable for the balance and quality of what they produce. In this way the new organizational arrangements address the problem of resistance of organizations, and in particular of the clinical staff, to new policies and objectives. The power to determine the product mix lies with the purchaser which, again in theory at least, should be more trustworthy in its pursuit of societal objectives than providers on a free rein. Culyer has named this 'demand side socialism'.

The purchaser / provider split has also brought out the planning role of the health authorities or purchasers. Although planning has been traditionally regarded as part of their function, the introduction of contracting places new emphasis on the purchaser's planning responsibility, as well as on a more explicit linkage between financing and the planning process. In order to set contracts purchasers are required to assess needs, establish priorities and to ensure that the most appropriate interventions are available to meet those needs within limited resources - in other words to plan. Despite 20 years of a formal NHS planning system, it was not until the introduction of contracting that well-recognized planning issues such as needs assessment and priority setting began to be taken seriously. Now, studies on priorities and needs assessment are flooding the NHS research agenda, and although planning seems to be a taboo word in the new NHS management culture, that is what the newly formed service development and contracting teams are actually doing. And now contracts provide what was the missing link between priorities and finance.

It can be argued that contracting implies a drastic 'zero based' approach to planning, according to which all existing health care services have to be comprehensively reviewed every contracting period to determine whether or not they should continue, at what scale, and with what level of resource use. The infeasibility of this approach was promptly recognized by the NHS management executive which affirmed that

"DHAs will not have the resources (staff, skills) to carry out the work necessary to lead informed change to the same degree in more than a limited number of areas"(NHSME, 1991).

In planning terminology this is the `mixed scanning' approach, in which each year a few priority areas are picked out for review and change, leaving the rest fundamentally as they stand (NHSME, 1991).

It seems that PB has been 'rediscovered' and is being discussed again in the context of the NHS (Bramley, 1993; Craig, 1993). Some purchasing units in the NHS are already working - perhaps without recognising it — within a 'PB framework', assessing needs, establishing priorities and contracting services for particular client or disease groups.

Overall, the introduction of contracting into the NHS has given a new emphasis to planning with more explicit priority setting and trade offs between competing needs and facilitating of the implementation of plans. However, its potential as a mechanism for the pursuit of planning objectives will depend on how it is operationalised.

THE CONTRACT AS A FINANCIAL MECHANISM FOR IMPLEMENTING PLANS

A contract can be seen as a financial mechanism for reimbursing the provider for an established set of services, who in exchange will be accountable for the delivery of these services. There is nothing intrinsically better than any other method of funding about adopting contracting for health service financing; its success in implementing planning objectives and ultimately in achieving allocative efficiency will depend on the financial method adopted, on how the services are specified and the effectiveness of its provision for monitoring and accountability.

In principle, the contracting potential for planning resides in its prospective nature and in specifying the services in terms of the quantity, mix and price of the outputs to be produced. First, a contract can serve as a vehicle for fixing the quantity and mix of health care products to be provided. Arguably, this combination will lead to a state of allocative efficiency provided that the chosen mix reflects societal utilities and technical efficiency is assumed. Second, a contract can serve as a mechanism of fixing the price of health care products for hospital reimbursement, eg. payment of US Medicare hospitals based on Diagnostic Related Groups. This will encourage minimisation of costs below the rate of payment fixed and thus encourage technical efficiency. Third, contracting can serve as a basis for introducing provider markets. In theory this will provide an incentive for price competition and further pressure for technical efficiency.

The relevance of these for contracting in the NHS is analyzed in the next three sections on:

i)   types of contract and allocative efficiency;
ii) effect of prospective payment by case mix on technical efficiency and quality;

iii) effect of competition on technical efficiency and quality.

A fundamental issue is the choice of case mix measure to fix the balance of services to be provided and the incentives generated by reimbursement based on case mix.

TYPES OF CONTRACT AND ALLOCATIVE EFFICIENCY

The specification of contracts for goods and services can in principle include detailed requirements relating to:

- *access*   *eg.* the service should include access to general acute hospital services, an ITU, day surgery, an interpreter, etc.;
- *resource levels*   *eg.* the service should include at least x whole-time equivalent consultant orthopaedic surgeons;
- *organisation*   *eg.* there should be regular clinical audit meetings;
- *process*   *eg.* clinic cancellation rates should be less than x%, waiting for procedure x should be less than y weeks;
- *activity*   *eg.* there should be at least x hip replacement operations per year, at least y people screened for breast cancer;
- *indications*   *eg.* only those with hearing loss of greater than x Db should have surgery for glue ear;
- *coverage*   *eg.* the service should provide treatment for x% of the eligible cases of osteo-arthrosis of the hip this year;
- *outcome*   *eg.* at least x% of those seen with heart attacks should survive at least y days; x months after hip replacement more than y% should be weight bearing and less than z% should have died.

The three contract categories introduced by the NHS reform, have different potential for implementing objectives depending on how the services are specified.

In the early stages after the NHS reform, the most common type has been the *block contract*, in which the provider is paid an annual sum in instalments, in return for *access* for the purchaser's residents to a defined range of services (DoH, 1989). Refinements of block contracts involve fixing the levels of provision of *resources* in terms of beds or doctors, linked to particular specialities. These are relatively simple items to specify and monitor, but the approach gives no guarantee in itself that providers will treat the kinds of patients that the purchaser regards as being of the greatest priority, or treat them in a way that the purchaser regards as being effective or of good quality. Crucial decisions about the volume and nature of outputs to be produced stay on the provider side. Whilst this may be necessary with some forms of acute care such as A&E, for elective procedures block contracts offer little scope for using contracting in pursuit of policies and priorities. In practice, block contracts in the NHS have embodied a degree of volume control, termed in 'indicative levels'. This has lead to many units using up funds before the end of the financial period.

In *cost and volume contracts*, the provider receives a sum of money in return for treating an specified number of cases (DoH, 1989). Any additional work has to be subject to separate negotiation. The areas covered by this kind of contract may be highly selected, mainly in areas of particularly high or low priority and indeed, in the first two years of the NHS reforms this type has represented only a small proportion of all contracts. Fixing the volume of *activity* and nature of health care outputs to be produced in this way is a better than block contracting in terms of its potential for implementing plans and priorities. However, as Roberts argues, units will still have to prioritise between patients.

> "It is unlikely that purchasers, given the budgetary constraints under which they are trading, will contract for enough cases to meet the needs of the population. Patients may, thus, risk not getting treatment and purchasers may face political pressures to extend the services" (Roberts, 1993).

Refinements of cost and volume contracts could include specifications of *coverage*, which can be based on purchasers' priorities; specifications of *indications* to ensure that services are provided to the people most in need of them; and specifications of *outcome* to ensure that the services provided are as effective as they should be and needs are actually met. However the scope for such refinements is still very limited in the light of current medical knowledge and information systems.

In *cost per case contracts*, the purchaser agrees — prospectively or retrospectively - a price for the treatment of an individual patient (DoH, 1989). For example the traditional approach for contracting hospital services by private insurance in US is based on retrospective payment of full costs; hospitals are reimbursed for all expenses incurred in health care provision and the charges that they make. If wholly retrospective in this sense, with an open-ended commitment to pay whenever and wherever treatment occurs, the purchaser has no control over the number, nature and often the price of the outputs produced. This creates obvious incentives for inefficient behaviour by providers and patients and gives the purchaser no leverage in terms of the pursuit of policies and plans. In the context of the NHS reforms it means setting up contingency funds for extracontractural referrals, which otherwise can lead to overspending and jeopardise the purchaser's viability. However this is the only approach which allows the patient - or the GP on the patients behalf - a more or less unfettered right to choose the place and the time of treatment. It could thus be argued that the principles of individual patient choice and community choice - as expressed via the planning process — are in conflict.

A refinement of the cost per case approach involves a prospective agreement between purchaser and provider over costs. In some situations price and eligibility have to be agreed for a specific patient by negotiation between purchaser and provider before treatment begins. This has been used to ensure that candidates for surgery meet predetermined indications. However it is clearly not practicable for purchasers and providers to negotiate in this way for every patient treated. One way round this is to set costs at an average level for each type of patient involved, as in the American prospective payments systems for Medicare based largely on Diagnosis Related Groups (Schweiker, 1982). As used in the US, there is no prospective agreement about the mix of types of patients to be treated, and in this form there is little scope to the purchaser to implement priorities or plans.

EFFECT OF PROSPECTIVE PAYMENT BY CASE MIX CLASSIFICATION ON TECHNICAL EFFICIENCY AND QUALITY

It seems that the form of *cost and volume* contract best fills the role of a mechanism for implementing plans. However this raises a question of 'volume of what'? How is the desired balance of health care products or case-mix to be defined? And what are the effects on technical efficiency and quality of using a case mix measure as a basis for prospective payment?

One possibility is the system of Diagnosis Related Groups, or some adaptation of it. It is worth reviewing the US experience here to illustrate the possible effect of the adoption of such a system in the NHS as a basis for contracting. The objective of their use in the US is improved technical efficiency. By prospectively fixing the rate of payment, providers are encouraged to reduce their own average costs below the national average. The incentives generated in the NHS should be similar to those seen in the US, the main difference being that in the NHS the rate of reimbursement is based not on national average costs but on local costs as constrained by competition with other providers.

The main effect of introducing prospective payment in the US has been that in general the rate of increase of cost per case has been relatively low in the hospitals involved (Robinson, 1988). In those cases where cost per case has declined, the main contributory factor appears to be a significant decline in length of stay (Feder, 1987), different studies reporting reductions of between 9% and 12% (Guterman, 1986; Des Harnais,1987). There has also been a total decline in inpatient admissions which is attributed to a tendency for hospitals to be more selective, to pre-authorization before admission and to a shift of patients from inpatient to out-patient care (Culyer, 1990). It is argued that the reduction of length of stay has been offset by an increase in severity of case-mix, so that the reduction in total costs has been due to a relative decrease in total admissions (Carter, 1985). But overall the introduction of prospective payment systems (PPS) has been considered a success in terms of *cost* containment, halving the rate of inflation in Medicare patients.

However, there are concerns about the impact of PPS on the *quality* of care. The DRG classification assumes equal quality of care and health outcomes within a particular group. As a result of this, new forms of treatment which offer improved outcome but at higher cost appear to be inefficient and may be discouraged. Also some of the cost savings have been achieved by using cheaper inputs or earlier patient discharge, and these too can have an impact on quality (Culyer, 1988). (Certainly there has been a simultaneous increase in the number of outpatient and private patient visits, probably because both these areas are still paid by retrospective payment at 'full cost'). Prospective payment will

> "enhance efficiency only to the extent that patients are not adversely affected and that additional costs are not imposed on other suppliers such as primary care physicians or through cost shifting" (Culyer, 1990).

The evidence about the impact on quality of the introduction of DRG reimbursement is unclear and often contradictory (Des Harnais, 1987; Shortell, 1988; Sager, 1989). A number of confounding factors such as changes in the severity of the case mix or early discharges to other institutions have undermined most evaluation studies. Culyer considers that

> "without further detailed studies and in particular without evidence of post discharge mortality rates, the true impact on patient outcomes of cost containment remains unclear" (Culyer, 1990).

There seem to be good grounds for introducing measures of quality of patient outcome for each DRG.

Thirdly, there is the question of whether DRGs are *equitable* or fair. It is claimed that there are substantial variations in the severity of illness of patients within groups, and thus in their needs for resources (McMahon, 1986). This means that hospitals with more that their fair share of severely ill cases, such teaching hospitals and those in deprived areas, will be underfunded. It also means that there is a risk of adverse selection, through incentives for providers not to accept patients that are expected to generate relatively high costs given their DRG. To tackle this problem a number of refinements to DRGs have been suggested (HSMG, 1989; Freeman, 1991) and a number of alternative or supplementary case mix measures such as Disease Staging (Gonnella, 1984), Patient Management Categories (Young, 1984) and APACHE (Knaus, 1985). Although using some these measures can reduce the amount of variation within groups in terms of resources used, the underlying problem remains.

There are a number of problems of adopting DRGs as they stand for use in the NHS. There are slightly differences in the diagnostic classification used (ICD9 rather than ICD9CM) and deficiencies in the quality of coding, which lead to cases being assigned to incorrect DRGs or not being assigned at all (Jenkins, 1989; Sanderson, 1989). Also the fact that the DRG system was developed in US has raised doubts about the appropriateness of the resource weights involved (Jenkins,1990). As a result a new case mix system of 'health related groups' or HRGs (National Case-Mix Office, 1992), based on DRGs, has recently been developed for the UK. This will use more appropriate cost weights and can use ICD 9 and OPCS 4, the British classification of procedures.

These or similar problems are likely to occur in any health care system and should be taken into account whenever a case mix product is used for payment. However, the introduction of market competition is likely to produce additional incentives for providers to manipulate case mix statistics.

EFFECT OF COMPETITION ON TECHNICAL EFFICIENCY AND QUALITY

In evaluating the impact of contracting it is necessary to assess the competitive environment within which health services are provided. The main reason for adopting contracting in the NHS has been to facilitate the introduction of a competitive market for health care provision. The origin of these ideas lies in the work of an American economist, Alain Enthoven (Enthoven, 1985). The rationale underlying provider markets is that

"competition provides both an incentive structure for improving efficiency and a transmission mechanism for spreading it throughout the service" (Robinson, 1989).

In addition, competition is expected to foster entrepreneurship, increase innovation, enhance consumer choice and liberate the system from bureaucracy (Roberts, 1993). At the same time, public funding is retained to overcome the inequitable distribution of health care inherent in a system based on the individual's capacity to pay.

The 'resurrection' of the market in public health systems comes as a response to the failures of public intervention, which paradoxically was primarily justified by market failures. Thus, the introduction of provider markets raises some of the same issues as private markets. This closes an ideological 'circle' represented by: 'market - public intervention - market' and raises the same dilemma of 'whether' to regulate, 'what' and 'how'.

Although central funding will counteract some of the distributional problems of the market approach, the conditions of perfect competition required to achieve efficiency will be absent in a provider market. Health care products are usually far from being marketable goods. These are

"homogeneous and can be supplied by many alternative suppliers, information is shared among consumers, providers and purchasers; and standards are easily set and monitored" (Roberts, 1993).

The contestability of health care markets - or the costless entry to or exit from the market place - has been questioned by several authors. Roberts argues that the presence of large sunk costs and specific assets in health care will diminish the contestability of the market, hence not providing the discipline necessary to ensure efficiency. If the contracts involve large investments and specific assets as they do for high technology care,

"it may well be that those firms who do not win contracts initially will disappear and subsequent contracting will be between fewer parties" (Roberts, 1993).

In addition, the information problems and the difficulties in setting and monitoring standards in health care leaves ample room for providers to manipulate the market in their favour. They may use a number of strategies which can have adverse effects in terms of efficiency equity and quality of health care. There are incentives for:

i)   segmenting the market and concentrating on relatively profitable areas;

ii)   adverse selection denying access to the most expensive cases or shifting them to other carers;

iii) differentiating the products and biasing information (Enthoven, 1988).

Note that some of the perverse incentives provided by case mix reimbursement, discussed in the previous section, can be exacerbated by competition.

Most of the empirical evidence comes from the US where hospital competition has been studied. The evidence seems to suggest that the effects of competition have been the opposite of what was expected. Although at the beginning some provider markets experienced lowering of costs, these increased subsequently due to a reduction in competition[1] and the fact that competition was based on quality rather than on price. Furthermore, competition has lead to excess capacity and duplication of facilities (Scheffler, 1991). It may be that some of these problems are determined by the specific characteristics of competition in the US rather than by competition in itself. The keys are the absence of any effective budget constraint on consumers and on retrospective hospital reimbursement which encourages inefficient behaviour and non price competition.

In the UK, there is not yet enough evidence to evaluate the effects of competition in provider markets. Activity figures for its first year of operation have shown an increase in consultant episodes and outpatient attendances (NAHAT, 1992). These have been attributed to efficiency improvements (NHSME, 1992), but there are a number of alternative explanations which may also explain this phenomenon. In particular, it is argued that increased activity can be due to an increase in funding (Petchey, 1993) or, more worrying, due to provider opportunistic behaviour biasing information. Seng argues that increases in activity as measured by consultant episodes may be due to causes other than efficiency such as changing recording practices or increasing the numbers of patients transferred between consultants during a single admission (Seng, 1993). Finally, it should be pointed out that the scope of the provider market is still very limited with more than 75 per cent of the DHA contracts established with local district providers -DMUs and Trusts (NAHAT, 1992).

In general the success of provider markets will depend on the opportunistic behaviour of providers and on the measures and safeguards introduced by the third party to counteract perverse incentives. Regulation will involve the introduction of a wide range of standards for accreditation, registration and quality measures in general. However this approach will first have to confront yet unsolved issues of outcome measurement and substantial administrative costs may jeopardise any possible efficiency gains.

---

[1]The competition was reduced as in initial rounds several firms went out of business leaving fewer first and few new entrants to bid in subsequent rounds (Scheffler, 1991).

CONCLUSIONS

The introduction of contracting in the NHS has implied changes in the organization of the system (the split between purchaser and provider) and in the planning function. These changes address the problems of managing programmes across hierarchically run organizations and organizational resistance to programme implementation, by allowing programme budget holders to purchase services across primary, community and hospital care. Furthermore, the decentralization of service management brought about by contracting allows managers to introduce incentives and to increase provider participation in overcoming barriers to change. At the same time the purchaser / provider split increases the purchaser's power to determine the mix of health care products, forcing them to evaluate alternative objectives and strategies and to adopt explicit priorities. However it should be stressed that contracting is not the only way of achieving these desirable ends. They could also be achieved by management decentralization and by reforming hospital reimbursement systems with for example the introduction of management budgets by objectives, and through reform of providers payment systems including the introduction of incentives.

The major potential of contracting as a mechanism for planning lies in the programming and implementation stages of the process. Contracting involves the translation of planning objectives and strategies into programmes with specific targets, standards and budget allocations; and more importantly, the implementation of these programmes through the allocation of earmarked resources. Yet, the realisation of this potential depends on the purchasers ability to determine prospectively the nature, volume and price of health care outputs to be produced.

In general, contracting will result in:

i) increased allocative efficiency if the nature and volume of health products determined by the contract reflect soundly based planning choices;

ii) increased technical efficiency if the price established leads to minimization of costs without any negative impact on outcomes.

These are, however, interlinked with the issues — reviewed above — of finding appropriate ways of defining health care products. There are no ideal case mix systems and their use for payment is bound to leave some room for opportunistic manipulation by providers. Nonetheless we argue that the benefits of using a case mix system and ensuring an appropriate mix of health care products through financial mechanisms outweigh the problems. The way forward should be the development of better classifications of case mix and improvement in quality specifications.

A further approach to increasing technical efficiency through contracting is price competition in provider markets. However, there is still little evidence about the impact of introducing provider markets on societal objectives, and the verdict on the need to adopt them remains open. In the NHS the introduction of contracting has been mainly justified by the need to introduce provider competition, but we argue that the real positive impact of contracting lies in the way it addresses the planning predicament, and that this transcends whatever benefits (or, otherwise) may accrue from competition.

REFERENCES

Bramley, P. (1993). A framework for programme budgeting and commissioning at locality level in East Sussex. Joint meeting of the Health Economists' Study Group and the Faculty of Public Health Medicine. University of York.

Carter, G, Ginsgburg, P. (1985). The Medicare case mix index: medical practice changes, ageing and DRG creep. R-3292-HCFA The RAND corporation. Santa Monica.

Comision de Analisis y Evaluacion del Sistema Nacional de Salud (CAE) (1991). Informe y Recomendaciones (informe Abril). CAESNS, Madrid.

Craig, N. (1993). Tools for making purchasing decisions in District Health Authorities: the return of Programme Budgeting and Marginal Analysis. Joint meeting of the Health Economists' Study Group and the Faculty of Public Health Medicine. University of York.

Culyer, A.J. (1988). Working Party on Alternative Delivery and Funding of Health Services. Working paper No 3. IHSM, London.

Culyer AJ, Posnett JW. (1990). Hospital Behaviour and Competition. In: Culyer AJ, Maynard AK, Posnett JW, eds. Competition in Health Care: Reforming the NHS. Macmillan, London.

Des Harnais, S, Kobrinski, E, Chesney, S, et al. (1987). The early effects of the prospective payment system on inpatient utilization and the quality of care. Inquiry, 24, 7-16.

DHSS (1976a). The NHS planning system. HMSO, London.

DHSS (1976b). Priorities for health and personal social services. HMSO, London.

DHSS (1977) 'The way forward'. HMSO, London.

DHSS (1983). NHS Management inquiry (Griffiths report). HMSO, London.

DoH. (1989). Funding and Contracts for Hospital Services. Working for Patients: Working paper 2. HMSO, London.

DoH (1990). National Health Service and Community Care Act. HMSO, London.

Enthoven, AC. (1985). Reflections on the Management of the National Health Service. Occasional Papers 5. Nuffield Provincial Hospitals Trust, London.

Enthoven, AC. (1988). Managed competition of alternative delivery systems. Journal of Health Politics, Policy and Law, 13, 305-320.

Feder, J, Hadley, J, Zuckerman, S. (1987). How did Medicare's prospective payment system affect hospitals? New England Journal of Medicine, 317, 867-73.

Freeman, JL. (1991). Refined DRGs: trials in Europe. Health Policy, 17, 151-164.

Glennerster, H. (1983). Planning for priority groups. Martin Robertson, London.

Gonnella, JS, Goran, MJ. (1984). Staging of a disease: a case-mix measurement. Journal of the American Medical Association, 251, 637-44.

Guterman, S, Dobson, A. (1986). Impact of the Medicare prospective payment system for hospitals. Health Care Financing Review, 7, 97-114.

Health Systems Management Group (1989). DRG refinement with diagnosis specific comorbidities and complications: a synthesis of current approaches to patient classification. Final Report. Yale University: Health Systems Management Group.

Jenkins, L, McKee, M, Sanderson, H. (1989). Problems of allocating patients to DRGs using UK data. In Diagnostic Related Groups (DRGs). NWTRHA. Regional Information Unit, London.

Jenkins, L, McKee, M. (1990). DRGs a guide to grouping and interpretation. CASPE Research, London.

Jones, T, Prowle, M. (1987). Health Service Finance. Certified Accountants Educational Trust, London.

Knaus, WA, Draper, EA, Wagdner, DP, Zimmerman, JE. (1985). APPACHE II: a severity of disease classification system. Crit. Care Med., 13, 818-29.

McMahon, L. Newbold, R. (1986). Variation in resource use within diagnosis-related groups. Medical Care, 24, 5, 388-397.

National Association of Health Authorities and Trusts. (1992). The financial survey 1992. NAHAT, Birmingham.

National Case-Mix Office (1992). Health Related Groups (HRGs). National Case-Mix Office, Winchester.

NHS Management Executive (1991). Moving Forward - Needs, Services and Contracts. A DHA Project Paper. HMSO, London.

NHS Management Executive. (1992). The NHS reforms; the first six months. HMSO, London.

Oxford English Dictionary. Volume II, C. Oxford University Press. 1933-

Packwood, T et al. (1991). Hospitals in transition. The resource management experiment. Open University Press, London.

Petchey, R. (1993). NHS Internal Market 1991-92: towards a balance sheet 306, 699-706.

Rathwell, T. (1987) Strategic planning in the health sector. Croom Helm, London.

Rea, C. (1992). 'Gang Mentality'. Health Service Journal. 26 March 1992, 31-34.

Roberts, JA. (1993). Managing markets. London: London School of Hygiene and Tropical Medicine. Journal of Public Health Medicine, December 1993 (forthcoming).

Robinson, J, Luft, H. (1988). Competition, regulation and hospital costs 1982 to 1986. Journal of the American Medical Association, 260, 2676-81.

Robinson, R. (1989). New health care market. BMJ 298, 437-9.

Rodwin, V. (1984). The Health Planning Predicament: France, Quebec, England and the United States. University of California Press.

Sager, MA, Easterling, DV, Kinding, DA, Anderson, OW. (1989). Changes in the location of death after passage of Medicare's Prospective Payment system. New England Journal of Medicine, 320, 433-39.

Saltman, RB, Von Otter, C. (1992). Planned Markets and Public Competition. Strategic Reform in Northern European Health Systems. Buckingham: Open University Press.

Sanderson, HF. (1989) Evaluation of Diagnosis Related Groups in the Resource Management project. Wessex RHA.

Scheffler, R, Nauenberg, E. (1991). Health care financing reform in the United States during the 1980's: Lessons for Great Britain. In McGuire, A, Fenn, P, Mayehew, eds. Providing health care. The economics of alternative systems of finance and delivery. Oxford University Press.

Schweiker RS. (1982). Hospital prospective payment for Medicare. Report to Congress. Washington: Department of Health and Human Services.

Seng, C, Lessof, L, McKee, M. (1993). Who's on the fiddle. Health Service Journal, 7 January 1993, 16-17

Shortell, SM, Hughes, EF. (1988). The effects of regulation competition, and ownership on mortality rates among hospital inpatients. New England Journal of Medicine, 318, 1100-07.

Wynand, PMMM. (1989). A future for Competitive Health Care in the Netherlands. NHS White paper. Occasional Paper 9. University of York: Centre for Health Economics.

Young, WW. (1984). Incorporating severity of illness and co-morbidity in case mix measurement. Health Care Financing Review, (supplement), 23-31.

17 Changing Patterns of Care — The Challenges for Health Care Professions and Professionals

CHARLES E.M. NORMAND

London School of Hygiene and Tropical Medicine

BACKGROUND

This paper explores the implications of changes in medicine and health care for health care professions and professionals. In particular it is concerned with changes that will occur as health services attempt to meet the aspirations of the populations. It also suggests some changes that might retain much of what is best in current patterns as circumstances change.

The changing face of medicine and health care has been widely explored in recent years [1,2]. The themes are familiar: biomedical science is expanding rapidly, technologies are developing, the patterns of diseases in the population are changing and the ageing population requires new patterns of services. Countries are exploring ways to address these opportunities and meet the financial implications [3]. There are challenges resulting from the present pattern of services. The inappropriate balance between primary and secondary care, and the need to provide better support for those requiring services for continuing and chronic conditions results in a need for investment in buildings, staff skills and equipment. Long lead times make planning facilities and staff difficult. The history of planning human resources for health in the United Kingdom has not been happy [4].

As in most production of goods and services, there is widespread inefficiency in the use of health sector resources. Some results from interventions which have little or no useful effect. Only around 15% of medical interventions are based on treatments that have been subjected to rigorous scientific testing [5]. Much of the rest is probably effective, but it is difficult to establish whether it is sufficiently useful to justify the resources used. Some is ineffective. Uncertainty about the effectiveness of many interventions is highlighted by the wide variation in the rates of treatments within countries and between countries [6,7]. Although the extent of inefficiency in

Managerial Issues in the Reformed NHS. Edited by M.Malek, P.Vacani, J.Rasquinha & P.Davey
© 1993 John Wiley & Sons Ltd

generating health gain is unknown, it is likely that significant improvements are possible within existing resources.

Inefficiency also exists in the production processes themselves. There are many choices between combinations of buildings, equipment, consumables and staff. For example, more sophisticated monitors allow fewer staff to be employed in observation of patients. The use of minimally invasive surgery may increase theatre time, but require less nursing staff and fewer beds. Many interesting issues are about substitution between staff groups, combinations of skills within professions, and the effects of professions on the delivery of health care.

HEALTH CARE AS A PRODUCTION PROCESS

To treat health care as a production process is not to deny many special characteristics; providing health care is not like making soap. However, for the purposes of exploring characteristics of the processes of health care production it is useful to draw on the industrial analogy.

Health care facilities have many products. Inputs of staff, equipment, facilities and consumables are combined in various ways to produce various products. This makes it difficult to apportion the activity of different staff and costs to the different products. For example, a doctor may be on-call for paediatrics, providing cover for emergencies in all parts of the service, and being actually present in the neonatal intensive care unit. This is one reason why our understanding of production processes is poor, and research into health services professionals so difficult[8].

Changes in medical technology lead to changes in what are efficient methods of producing health services. The obvious manifestations of this are new techniques and devises, such as angioplasty, lithotrypsy and minimally invasive surgery. However, possibly more important than changes in the availability of equipment are changes in ideas. There is a case for describing such developments as technological change[9]. Shorter lengths of stay, discharge of people with learning difficulties to care in the community and hospice care are partly understandable as changes in ideas, and are as such changes in health care technology. The idea of patient focused care and the patient focused hospital are examples of this type of change. Ideas offer the greatest potential for achieving more efficient production of health services. The persistence of old ideas can be a constraint.

The mix of staff and other inputs into production of health care can and does vary. The most vivid examples are in international comparisons of health care provision[10]. For example, the ratio of nurses to doctors is around 1 in Portugal and 5 in Ireland. Hospital admission rates in France are nearly double those of the Netherlands. Despite the clear evidence of there being choices in the mix of inputs into the production process, the idea of factor substitution has not been applied widely in the analysis of health care production. Many planning decisions for hospital services use ratios to determine the need for different inputs. Labour displacing technology is introduced without displacing labour, and machines designed to be substitutes are often used in parallel. When changes do occur they are often very large and sudden[11].

Much of the inefficiency from a failure to adapt is pure waste (X-inefficiency)[12]. Some is from using the wrong mix of factors or ignore inputs altogether, such as the use of private cars for access, or the time of informal carers. One effect of this is to overstate the existence of economies of scale in the provision of health services[13]. Reasons for inefficiency in the production of health services include incentives, limited information, market failure and constraints and controls on health care staffing. Most of this paper is devoted to analysis of staffing and professional issues.

PROFESSIONS AND HEALTH CARE

Professions have many rôles. The justification for allowing restrictive practices and monopoly power is that there are countervailing benefits of safety and quality of services. For operational purposes it can be useful to define a profession by the fact that members have responsibilities through a body of knowledge to the profession (and therefore the client) as well as to the employer. In other words, some actions desired by the professional or employer are prescribed by the profession. Some of these have resource consequences. Rules mainly concern the conduct of the work, but may also include fees charged and other economic interests.

Explicit licensing and controls exist for most professions, but in addition there are often professional standards to encourage improvement in the quality of interventions. There is no single idea of what is the basis for professional standards. In a recent study three different interpretations were evident[14]. These are quite illuminating since they emphasise the potential for the rôle of professions to be useful or harmful. The first of these is that standards should be what would be done in the absence of recourse constraints. While being of little value in terms of an aspiration, such a concept can be helpful in providing a datum point against which actual standards can be compared. However, economists would argue that achieving such standards is undesirable, since higher priority uses of the resources must necessarily exist.

At the opposite extreme professional standards can be conceived of as a floor below which it is better not to provide the intervention. Although this does not define the most desirable pattern of provision, it is useful as a guide to when no treatment may be the preferred option. It can also be helpful in identifying the core and essential components of an intervention. This notion of standards has the disadvantage that pressure can develop to take this minimum cost option as the standard. The third concept of professional standards is less easily described since it lacks fixed or absolute characteristics. Professional standards are best understood as part of a process of change. The idea is to effect improvements in service quality, and the process involves setting standards higher than present practice. Insofar as current practice can be improved without resource consequences this is unobjectionable. However, if additional resources are required, it is not necessarily the best use of these resources.

Professional standard setting and attempts to meet such standards can therefore be seen as potentially useful, but also potentially harmful. The important point is that professionals may reduce the value of health gain from a given level of resources *even when their behaviour is disinterested.* Taking a holistic view of resources and the quality, quantity and mix of services provided, professional standards that increase the resources and quality for a single intervention may increase or decrease health gain. Interested behaviour by professions can reduce health gain in several ways. Successful action to increase salaries reduces the effective budget, and restrictive practices can reduce competition and therefore raise costs. For the purposes of the argument here the first is not of interest. However, professional boundaries, defining tasks and skills associated with particular professions can seriously reduce the scope for improving the quantity and quality of health care.

ISSUES IN THE FUTURE OF PROFESSIONS

There is no sense in which the argument in this paper rejects the notion of professions or challenges their future existence. What does need careful analysis is how the advantages of professions and professionalism can be combined with the need to provide appropriate health services at minimum cost. Reasons why professions may prevent this are constraints on skill mix, failure to effect factor substitution where this is appropriate and constraints on team work. There are also some questions about the appropriateness of multiple levels of professions. For example, pathologists, surgeons and consultants in communicable disease control are all controlled as professionals at the level of being doctors as well as at the specialist level.

The mix of skills needed to provide a particular service can require many different professionals to be involved, although some of them play only a small part. Bundles of skills are grouped together into professions in ways that reflect historical developments. The somewhat arbitrary nature of these groupings can be seen when international comparisons are made[15]. Distinctions between the therapy professions are best understood in terms of history. For example (and similar examples are available for other professions) occupational therapists carry out a range of interventions from identifying the need for home modifications for people with physical handicaps to therapeutic interventions for children with mental health problems. Either of these could logically be located within another profession.

Combining skills into fairly rigid sets has obvious resource implications, since much of the training received is irrelevant or actually harmful. To justify a professional organisation there must be a significant content to the skills, and this can be achieved either by having high level skills over a narrow range or a wider range of lower level skills. The latter will tend to leave unused many skills acquired at considerable cost. Left unused many skills disappear. The debate about the boundaries of the rôles of nurses and doctors reflects a desire to hold onto tasks that could well be performed by others for fear of undermining the medical profession[16].

This concern is made more relevant by the fact that many tasks traditionally carried out by doctors can in fact be provided adequately by other professionals.

Besides the waste of training resources, boundaries between professions can be harmful in terms of the quality of the experience of being a patient. There is wide consensus that patients should not be asked to interact with many health care staff, since this leads to confusion, repetition of assessments and data collection, and a difficulty in giving the care a patient focus. The implication of this is that different care activities really require bespoke bundles of skills in each of the staff, which combine to cover all the necessary competencies. Some duplication and reserves are needed since some will be needed throughout the 24 hours, and are sensibly available in various combinations. The logic of this is that at least some types of professionalism need to be in a modular framework, with competencies being defined, and a selection of such competencies being gained by any individual. Service providers would aim to employ people with the most appropriate mixtures. Skills could be assembled over time by staff. A structure such as formal national vocational qualifications (NVQ and Scotvec) could be adapted to insure standards.

The approach to skill mix of staff and care teams outlined above leaves difficulties for professions and professional identity. One reason for the ability of professions to impose standards and responsibilities on members is that they can exploit the loyalty of professionals to the profession. For example, the tasks of mental handicap nurses in the care of people with learning difficulties owe little in terms of process to general nursing, and similarly nurses working in theatre use few general nursing skills. However, there are some attitudes and ethical positions that they all share, many of which have a useful rôle in developing good quality care. This also applies to some other staff, who lack professional qualifications, but take their working identity from nursing. Logic might see the development of the idea of professionalism in health care, with caring and ethical principles shared by all. Retention of professionalism in a world of diverse mixes of skills in health care workers might be difficult.

If the move towards skills development outlined above were to take place, and there are several settings in which there are early signs, a major question is the way that medical professions would fit in. Several factors potentially cause problems. First, doctors are normally treated as quite separate from other professionals, and there is a large difference in the expected career development and financial rewards. Training of doctors normally follows separate routes, with structures that make it difficult to transfer into medicine from the other health professions. Little or no allowance is made for learning or skills that have developed before entry into medical training. It is a subtlety of many professions that a barrier to entry into membership can be the requirement to engage in low level specific training before advancing (a slight exception to this is the exemption from up to one year of medical training for people with science or nursing backgrounds). This is expensive and time consuming, and can deter entry.

Logic would dictate that, if health professionals develop their skills through competencies that can be combined to provide a basis for a range of interventions, then such a route should allow access to some of the rôles and functions of the medical profession. It has long been recognised in the UK that the training of doctors has to change to recognise changes in health care practice, and the need for significant amounts of training beyond the basic qualification[17, 18, 19].

An argument against delegation of tasks traditionally carried out by doctors to other health care professionals is that medical training is more rigorous, has a stronger basis in the basic sciences, and therefore can equip the practitioner to identify the unexpected and unusual, and to take an analytical and sceptical position. There is some force in this argument, but it is not clear that the difference in the depth and rigour is now very great between, for example, the science base of general medical training and that of the new nursing training under Project 2000[20]. More to the point, it is not clear that the often didactic and knowledge based teaching really prepares doctors for a distinct rôle.

None of this argument should be taken to challenge the need for the equivalent of the specialist and general medical practitioners who are involved in highly complex and skilled interventions. It does, however, question whether the route taken to this licensed practice is particularly sensible. Put another way, what is the significance of the basic medical qualification if it has ceased to be a licence to do anything without supervision. In the UK the attainment of higher training qualifications, accreditation and consultant posts are all of much greater significance than the basic qualification. Two examples may be helpful. In Italy, the profession of dentistry has only recently been an option without a prior qualification in medicine. In countries with a tradition of independent dentistry this seems odd. France does not recognise a non medical profession of optometry, and the work of optometrists is taken by ophthalmologists. Eastern and central Europe has displayed many cases of rôles that have ceased to be restricted to medical personnel in the West, such as environmental health officers and hospital managers[21]. There is no reason why some of these development should not occur in more 'core' areas of medical practice, such as in surgery, control of communicable diseases and cardiology. Some confusion of rôles already exists in the dividing line between health psychologists, psychiatrists and psychiatric nurses, and the logic of requiring a medical qualification for psychotherapy is quite unclear. Midwives, obstetricians and general practitioners have heavily overlapping rôles in ante-natal care.

It is argued above that the medical qualification *per se* has ceased to have a great relevance, and may indeed be a constraint to the provision of appropriate training for specialised rôles. The logic of moves towards team working means that the full set of skills comes from the team, working in a mutually supportive way. Whilst team leadership is important, it is not self evident that the best team work comes when one profession is always leader. The end of the idea of a medical qualification may help to encourage other health care professionals to take on leadership rôles.

Of all branches of medicine, general practice comes closest to being the application of the content of the basic medical qualification, although further training is necessary and is now required. The skill of general practitioners (GPs) is to apply intermediate level competencies across a wide range of interventions. Under this scenario the training of GPs might be quite close to the present medical training, although there are some areas in which much more emphasis is needed, most obviously in prescribing and mental health. However, another way of looking at the training of GPs is that it is peculiarly suited to being the accumulation of modules of competencies, since some skill is needed in a range of branches of medicine and health care.

The attempt in this section has been to follow through the effects of the changing needs of health services for skills, and identify the implications for the types of professions needed, and the ways in which these might be created. It is not suggested that the predicted trends will lead to rapid or obvious short term changes in licensing and training of staff, but that the present arrangements are unstable, and some of the current professional monopolies will be eroded. The future for health care professions is likely to be less tidy, with larger numbers of people with ranges of skills and levels of skills which fit badly into the present structures. If this happens there is a need for new and innovative ways to make use of the benefits of professionalism in medical practice, ensure competence, assure quality of care and to create coherent careers for health care staff.

IMPLICATIONS FOR POLICY

The objective of health services providers is to provide high quality, safe and cost-effective health services for their population, and for this they need skilled and motivated staff. There is good evidence that the detailed circumstances of the employment of staff are important in the morale of staff, and in the ability of employers to recruit and retain staff. Recent research suggested that at least half of the variation in turnover rates across the country is related to the characteristics of the job, and not the wider labour market[22]. Even in areas of low unemployment and many other opportunities to work outside the health service it is possible to recruit and retain staff. It is therefore important to ensure that any changes in the basis of employing staff takes this into account. Drawing on professionalism and treating staff as professionals seems to be an important part of job satisfaction in the health sector. There is a need to continue to define skilled staff in these terms.

With professions defined in broader terms, with more focus on the universal values and standards their focus will be the mission and of care agenda, and not specific sets of skills. As what is currently seen as cross training (ie the training of a professional in skills normally associated with another profession) becomes more widespread, there is a need to ensure that professionalism in these new tasks is maintained.

An important area for policy development is in the licencing of health care professionals. A more flexible system is needed, allowing several routes into practice of the advanced level skills. Professions must adapt to the changing trands and needs in health services risk decline and possible elimination. Change may be slow and evolutionary, but the benefits of professionalism will be lost if the present boundaries remain as care patterns change. New structures will need to be looser and more flexible to accommodate the changes in technology, and the consequent changes in care patterns. For team work to work, distinctions in status will have to be less, and more varied bundles of skills accommodated.

REFERENCES

1   Beck E, Lonsdale S, Newman S and Patterson D (eds) (1992) *In the best of health: the status and future of health care in the UK* London: Chapman and Hall

2   Smith R (ed) (1992) *The future of health care* London: BMJ Publishing

3   Normand C (1992) Funding Health Services in the United Kingdom. *British Medical Journal* 304:768-70

4   Birch S, Maynard A, Walker A   (1986)   *Doctor manpower planning in the United Kingdom: problems arising from myopia in policy making* York: Centre for Health Economics Discussion Paper no 18, University of York

5   Smith R (1991) Where is the wisdom? The poverty of medical evidence *British Medical Journal* 303:798-799

6   McPherson K   (1993)   Diversity and similarity of health: organisation, practice and assessment   in Normand C and Vaughan P (eds)   *Europe without Frontiers: the implications for health* Chichester: John Wiley and Sons

7   Wennberg J E, Freeman J L and Culp W J (1987) Are hospital services rationed in New Haven or over-utilised in Boston *Lancet* 1: 1185-1189

8   Phillips VL, Gray AM, Hermans D and Normand C (1992) *Health and Social Services Manpower in the UK: a review of research 1986-92* London: PHP Publication No 7, London School of Hygiene and Tropical Medicine ISSN:0962-6115

9   Uttley S (1991) *Technology and the welfare state* London: Unwin Hyman

10 Figueras J, Normand C, Roberts J et al (1991) *Health Infrastructure Needs of the Lagging Regions* Report to the Commission of the European Communities, London: London School of Hygiene and Tropical Medicine

11 Taylor B and Kelly T   (1990) *Outpatients departments: changing the skill mix.* A study conducted by the NHSME VFM Unit   London: HMSO

12 Leibenstein H   (1966)   Allocative efficiency versus X-efficiency *American Economic Review* 56: 397-409

13 Normand C (1991) Economics, Health and the Economics of Health   *British Medical Journal* 303; 1572-1577

14 Normand C, Ditch J, Dockrell J et al (1991)   *Clinical audit in professions allied to medicine and related therapy professions*   Report to the Department of Health Belfast: The Queen's University of Belfast, Health and Health Care Research Unit

15 McKee CM, Clarke A, Kornitzer et al (1992) Public health medicine training in the European Community: is there scope for harmonisation *European Journal of Public Health* 2: 45-53

16 McKee CM and Lessof L (1992) Nurse and doctor: whose task is it anyway? in Robinson J, Gray AM and Elkan R (eds) *Policy issues in nursing* Milton Keynes, Open University Press

17 Lowry S (1993) Trends in health care and their effects on medical education *British Medical Journal* 306: 255-258

18 Medical Committee of University Funding Council (1991) *First report of the effects of the NHS reforms on medical and dental education and research* London: UFC

19 Medical Committee of University Funding Council (1992) *Second report of the effects of the NHS reforms on medical and dental education and research* London: UFC

20 United Kingdom Central Council for Nursing, Midwifery and Health Visiting (1986) *Project 2000: A new preparation for practice* London, UKCC

21 McKee CM, Bojan F and Normand C (on behalf of the Tempus Consortium for a new Public Health in Hungary) (1993) A New Programme for Public Health Training in Hungary *European Journal of Public Health* 3:58-63

22 Gray AM and Phillips VL (1992) *Explaining NHS staff turnover: a local labour market approach* Report to the Department of Health. London, Health Services Research Unit, London School of Hygiene and Tropical Medicine

18 NHS Reform — The Final Frontier?

MO MALEK, PAUL VACANI & JOE RASQUINHA

University of St. Andrews

The N.H.S. reforms introduced in 1989 were the most radical set of changes introduced since inception of the organisation in 1948. Reorganising a massive institution and remoulding it into a newly restructured model inevitably involves costs — emotional, transitional, managerial and others, this begs the question that these changes were:

(i)   necessary
(ii)   cost-effective

Before the introduction of the reforms the N.H.S. was widely believed to be the major 'British' model of success, in terms of organisation, cost, quality and output. In short, a workable, value for money solution well worth emulating. The fact that other industrialised nations also seemed to have suddenly concerned themselves with the reform of their health services seemed to be irrelevant. This was because the health expenditure per capita in the UK was at the lower end of the league table Table 1), and the general consensus was that the health of the nation was not suffering from this at all.

The all intriguing question of 'if it is not bust why fix it' was answered in terms of the ideological imperatives of the new right. Whose preoccupation with dismantling of the welfare state, and all that which smacked of socially provided mass consumption, with the eventual aim of the privatisation of health care provision in Britain. Undoubtedly there is some element of truth in this. There is also a fact that the N.H.S., despite being value for money (in comparison with other industrialised countries), health expenditures (or at least their rate of growth) were of concern to the Conservative government because of the long term poor performance of the British economy.

Whatever the real motive behind the reform package may have been, the academic discourse revolved around the merits of markets and competition in achieving the goals of the government policy. Surprisingly, the objectives of government policy has remained unchanged. Infact The Griffiths Report was at pains to point out that delivering universal health care free of charge at the point of delivery, was still the

Managerial Issues in the Reeformed NHS. Edited by M.Malek, P.Vacani, J.Rasquinha & P.Davey
© 1993 John Wiley & Sons Ltd

Country	1960	1970	1980	1984
Canada	5.5	7.2	7.3	8.4
France	4.3	6.1	8.5	9.1
Germany	4.7	5.5	7.9	8.1
Italy	3.9	5.5	6.8	7.2
Japan	3.0	4.4	6.4	6.6
U.K.	3.9	4.5	5.6	5.9
U.S.A.	5.3	2.6	9.5	10.7

Table 1. Total Health Care Expenditure in Selected OECD Countries;
1960 — 1984 (Percent of GDP)
Source: OECD, *Financing and Delivery Health Care*, Paris 1987, Table 18.

main goal of health policy[4]. Looking through the vast amount of literature produced since then, it is clear that there are three criteria against which the success or failure of the regime should be judged. These are *efficiency, equity* and *cost containment*. These, together with the managerial background to the reforms, are discussed below.

EFFICIENCY

The object of efficiency, in its broadest interpretation, involves not only cost control, but also effectiveness. The need to 'do the right things and do the things right'. This was mainly to be achieved through 'managed competition' or as Alan Maynard puts it (quite correctly since it deals with the supply side only) 'regulated competition'[5]. In this process the position of the end users (patients) remained unchanged and the same agency relationship between the doctors and patients prevailed as before. The 'consumer choice' in this context was probably the red herring and the mechanism through which this choice had to be exercised, as well as the extent to which the choice had expanded was practically irrelevant. However, the purchaser-provider division and the contracting mechanism was to bring competitive forces into play, force down prices and increase output, thus bringing about a more efficient allocation of resources.

The premises upon which the smooth working of this 'social market' were based were rather dubious, not only because of the peculiarity of 'health care' as a commodity, but also because the necessary condition for product competition, is that competing products should be comparable with regards to price and/or quality, a condition which in this case would be very difficult to fulfil.

The information base of the N.H.S. prior to the reform was very poor indeed. This was probably expected from a highly bureaucratised, public monopoly. Prior to the reforms in the managerial structure and organisation of the N.H.S. there was very little need for such information. However, the situation changed drastically after the reforms as contracting became the central feature of the new structure. Information was needed with regards to costs, prices, quality, output and productivity of provider units, not only to facilitate transactions between purchasers and providers, but also to prevent underhanded cross-subsidisation.

EQUITY

It is not all that easy to ascertain the precise notion of equity adopted by the N.H.S. This ambiguity creates some problems, because each notion carries a different ideological weight and has different policy implications[1]. It seems to be the case that equality of access (and not utilisation) has been and remains, post reform, the principle equity objective behind the N.H.S. As such, in theory there is no *a priori* reason to believe that the post-reform N.H.S. will be less equitable. Since the financing method by general taxation has remained unchanged, it really is a matter of empirical evidence to establish whether the new system is more or less equitable.

COST CONTAINMENT

The following four reasons are among those most often cited for escalating health expenditure in industrialised countries:

(i) The grouping of population i.e. the age structure of the population growing older, people living longer and hence needing more healthcare. Presently more than a third of total health expenditure is spent on the care of the elderly;
(ii) Introduction of new more expensive medical technology;
(iii) The arrival of new epidemics like HIV/AIDS;
(iv) High income elasticity of demand of health.

If we accept these premises (which we should not), a cursory look at these factors reveals nearly all (except perhaps the new technology which is exogenously determined) are driven by demand. On the other hand, the nature of the N.H.S. reforms is to regulate the supply side and in this context there is very little scope for cost containment. To put it another way, supply efficiencies are a one off type efficiency, once one moves from inside the Production Possibility Frontier (PPF) to the curve, any increase in output has to be accompanied by an increase in the budget (see Figure 1).

Of course it is possible that managerial and organisational development leads to a further movement of the PPF, but again this is not a continuous movement and eventually will come to a halt.

The whole idea of *efficiency gain* through competition among providers is also a dubious one, because the nature of the market is that even if prices are set properly, real competition will be shifted from the cost/price side to the domain of quality, (a very valuable lesson to be learned from the private sector, especially the pharmaceutical industry). In this context competition will be cost increasing instead of cost decreasing.

A possible area of cost containment would be the use of economic evaluation techniques to compare and price alternative procedures, methods and so on. This has

Figure 1. Production Possibility Frontier

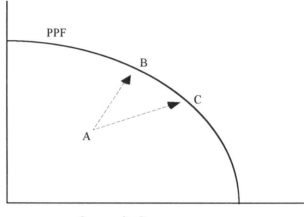

Technology
Intensive
Care

Community Care

the highest potential in terms of efficiency gains in production as well as consumption. However, like everything else this would be costly and requires an investment in terms of creating a data base and updating it and providing an appropriate network for dissemination of the information.

MANAGERIALISM V PROFESSIONALISM

Perhaps the most important aspect of the N.H.S. reforms were those which addressed the managerial issues and the resultant managerial structure of the health service. Griffiths' immortal words about Florence Nightingale having difficulty in finding who was in charge of the N.H.S. prior to the reform, must be one of the most cited quotations in recent times. There is no doubt that there has been some dislocation and re-distribution of power in the reformed N.H.S. The split in the purchaser-provider functions did create GP fundholders, although the power of medical profession has not reduced – yet. But the centre of gravity of power has substantially shifted from secondary cure consultants to the primary cure GPs who now have tremendous purchasing power.

It is sometimes asserted that the contamination of the power position of the medical profession was the price paid by Bevan to acquire their consent to introduce the N.H.S. The basis of this assertion is Bevan's quotation that he bought them (the consultants) by filling their mouths with gold. However, the truth is much more complicated than that and the power position occupied by the medical profession has a long history which goes back in history to before the middle ages, and the introduction of the N.H.S. merely formalised a social relationship which was already in place. Several attempts at reorganising the N.H.S. with the specific aim of introducing managerialism into the service, were tried and failed[8]. The only line of thought which could be consistently picked up about the management of the service was that it emphasised management by objective. The medical profession was present at each layer of the hierarchy with the power of veto eternally enshrined under the euphemism of 'clinical freedom', 'clinical autonomy', or similar.

At the area level local professional advisory committees, central health services councils and associated specialist sub-committees at regional level, and District Medical Committees at the district level (members of which sat on the District Management Team) were some of the formal channels of communication between the management and the professionals. In this context the power of managers was reduced to day to day running of functions which had already been decided, and it requires little exaggeration to claim that medicine was being *administered* rather than *managed*.

The Griffiths Inquiry and report spotted this rather weak link and sought to remedy the general management of the service. The recommendations placed emphasis on:

> " 1.   A satisfactory role at the centre with a split between policy making and implementation and the DHSS being reoriented to include in its broader activities support for the Supervisory Board and the Management Board.
>
> 2.   Delegation with hospitals free to take as many decisions as possible.
>
> 3.   Involvement of professionals in the management process.
>
> 4.   On a consideration as to what service the N.H.S. should provide.
>
> 5.   Determination of objectives; measurement of output; clinical and economic evaluation of work.
>
> 6.   Concern for the best deal for patients, staff and the taxpayer.
>
> 7.   On a general management role the essence of which is to improve accountability to seek major change and to secure motivation of staff.
>
> 8.   Need for the estate function to act in a more business like fashion.
>
> 9.   Need for a strong personnel function."[4]

The implementation of these recommendations involved tremendous financial costs yet a key instruction issued during the implementation of the report from Whitehall had been that there should be no overall increase in management costs[8].

The Griffiths recommendations and the reform package which was introduced in 1989 were revolutionising the whole structure of the health care together with its deep rooted culture and organisation. However, it was amazingly clear that despite a strong market rhetoric and blind faith in the working of the market, the package lacked the most basic ingredient, namely an incentive structure.

The reforms had released a wane of expectations among the most progressive managers. However, the word from Whitehall was to go as slowly as possible. Managers in 1991-92 were instructed to maintain a 'steady state' and then in 1992-93 to 'manage change' and be prudent. Despite all these, it seems that the managerial revolution has at last arrived in the N.H.S. with some irreversible results.

CONCLUSION

It is alleged that   Chou En-Lai was asked to give his opinion on the French Revolution of 1789 and he declined on the grounds that "it was still too soon". It certainly is too early to evaluate the consequences of the structural changes which have been brought about by the recent reforms. Proper assessments are a matter of empirical investigations and these have yet to materialise. From what has become available one can make few observations.

Firstly, the rather naive and outdated perception of the market, embodied in the reforms package, leaves few theoretical holes over the validity of the reforms and their comparative advantage over the alternatives, (which views markets as merely a network linking economic agents, which need it to communicate and adjust their output and prices). The new economic paradigm considers this to be only part (and at times not the most significant part) of the truth. Competition is important, but co-operative behaviour, customer relations, cultural background and expectations are also important.

It is probably wrong and premature to criticise the reformed N.H.S. for the massive investment expenditure in personnel and information technology[5]. Remembering that Sir Roy Griffiths, coming with a background of successful supermarket chains in which management costs are 13% (as compared to pre-reform N.H.S. which were approximately 5%) and the complex information requirement of the new management, these investments are probably justified. Any system undergoing such a structural change will inevitably have some transition costs, adjustment costs and costs involved with dealing with short-term bottlenecks. There are managerial problems that can not be predicted no matter how good the theoretical planning. Good managers understand pragmatism.

The most glaring shortcoming of the system seems to be its lack of a balanced mix of sanctions of incentives, performance indicators (quality assessment, quality control) and proper accountability above local level. This was brought to the public arena with the problems of fund mismanagement in the West Midlands and Wessex. One has to keep an open mind and regard this as an ongoing project.

The reforms are set to boldly go where no other reorganisation has attempted to go before. We need to read more from the Captain's logs before we are able to evaluate the new enterprise.

REFERENCES

1.   Brazier, J., Hutton, J., and Richard Jevons. *Evaluating the Reforms of the N.H.S.*, in
        Culyer *et al* (eds) (1990), pp 216 - 236.

2.   Culyer, A.J., Maynard, A.T., and Posnett, J.W. (eds). *Competition in Health Care*,
        MacMillan Press, 1990.

3.   DHSS (1983), N.H.S. Management Inquiry (Griffiths Report), HMSO, London.

4.   Griffiths, Sir Roy (1992), Seven Years of Progress - General Management in the NHS,
        Health Economics, Vol. 1, pp 61 - 70.

5.   Maynard, A., (1993), Competition in the UK National Health Service: Mission Impossible ?, *Health Policy*, Vol. 23, pp 193 - 204.

6.   OECD (1987), *Financing and Delivering Health Care*, Paris 1987.

7.   Office of Health Economics (1977), *The Reorganised NHS*, London.

8.   Strong, P., and Robinson, J., (1990), *The NHS Under New Management*, Open University Press, Milton Keynes.

Index

Index compiled by Liza Weinkove